EATING FOR TWO:
A GUIDE TO SAFE AND NUTRITIOUS CHOICES DURING PREGNANCY

Message From the Author

As a medical student, I have always been interested in promoting health and wellness. During my studies and clinical rotations, I have had the opportunity to work with pregnant women and have observed firsthand the challenges that they can face when it comes to understanding what they should and should not be eating during their pregnancy.

While there is a wealth of information available on this topic, it can be overwhelming and confusing for expectant mothers to try to sort through it all and make informed decisions about their diet. This motivated me to write a book on the topic, with the goal of providing a comprehensive and reliable resource for pregnant women.

I wanted to create a book that would cover all the essential nutrients that pregnant women need, as well as address common misconceptions and myths surrounding pregnancy nutrition. I believe that by empowering pregnant women with accurate and evidence-based information, we can support the health and well-being of both mothers and their babies.

In writing this book, I have drawn upon my medical education and research to ensure that the information provided is trustworthy and accurate. I have also included practical tips and guidance on how to incorporate the recommended foods into a healthy pregnancy diet.

I hope that my book will be a valuable resource for pregnant women and contribute to the promotion of optimal health outcomes for families. As a medical student, I am committed to promoting health and wellness in any way that I can, and I believe that by providing reliable information on pregnancy nutrition, I can make a positive impact on the lives of expectant mothers and their families.

Disclaimer

DISCLAIMER: The information contained in this book is intended for educational and informational purposes only. It is not intended as a substitute for professional medical advice, diagnosis, or treatment. If you have any concerns or questions about your health, you should always consult with a licensed healthcare professional. The author and publisher of this book are not responsible for any errors or omissions, or for any actions taken based on the information contained in this book. The author and publisher also make no representations or warranties with respect to the accuracy or completeness of the information contained in this book.

The information contained in this book is not intended to diagnose, treat, cure, or prevent any disease. The information is not intended to be a substitute for medical care provided by a licensed and qualified healthcare professional. The reader should consult with their healthcare provider in any matters relating to their health, and particularly in respect to any symptoms that may require diagnosis or medical attention.

The author and publisher of this book are not responsible for any adverse effects or consequences resulting from the use of any of the information contained in this book. The reader assumes all risks and liabilities associated with the use of the information contained in this book. The author and publisher do not endorse any specific products or treatments discussed in this book.

This book is not intended to create a physician-patient relationship between the reader and the author or publisher. The reader should be aware that the information contained in this book may not be suitable for everyone and should use their own discretion and judgment in determining the appropriateness of the information for their own situation. The reader should also be aware that the information contained in this book may not be applicable to their specific circumstances, and that the recommendations and advice provided may not be appropriate for their particular needs.

By reading this book, the reader agrees to indemnify and hold the author and publisher harmless from any damages or liabilities that may arise as a result of the use of the information contained in this book. The reader also agrees to waive any and all claims against the author and publisher, and to release the author and publisher from any and all liability for any injury or harm that may result from the use of the information contained in this book.

The author and publisher of this book are not responsible for the content of any third-party websites or resources that may be referenced or linked to in this book. The inclusion of any link does not imply endorsement by the author or publisher of the linked site or resource. The author and publisher are not responsible for the accuracy, completeness, or reliability of any information, data, opinions, advice, or statements contained on these third-party websites or resources. The reader should use their own discretion and judgment in relying on any information contained on these third-party websites or resources.

This disclaimer is subject to change without notice. The reader should review this disclaimer carefully before using the information contained in this book. By using the information contained in this book, the reader agrees to be bound by the terms of this disclaimer. If the reader does not agree to the terms of this disclaimer, they should not use the information contained in this book.

Preface

As an expectant mother, it can be overwhelming to navigate all the conflicting information out there about what is safe to eat and drink during pregnancy. That's where this book comes in – a sincere and supportive guide filled with reliable, up-to-date information to help you make informed decisions about your diet and lifestyle during this important time.

From common staples like caffeine and alcohol, to more unusual items like herbal supplements and certain types of fish, this book covers it all. But it's not just about what to avoid – we also include a wide range of safe and nutritious options for you to choose from. From healthy snacks to delicious and nourishing meals, you'll find plenty of ideas to help you and your baby get the nutrients you both need.

Whether you're a first-time mom or an experienced parent, this book has something for everyone. We understand that pregnancy can be a confusing and overwhelming time, and our goal is to provide you with the knowledge and support you need to make the best choices for you and your baby. We hope this book will be a helpful and reassuring resource for you during this special time.

Table of Contents

Tavsimran S. Luthra

EATING FOR TWO:
A GUIDE TO SAFE AND NUTRITIOUS CHOICES DURING PREGNANCY

Acetaminophen for pain relief

Acetaminophen is a pain reliever and fever reducer that is commonly used to treat mild to moderate pain. It is the active ingredient in many over-the-counter and prescription pain medications, such as Tylenol. Acetaminophen works by reducing the production of prostaglandins, which are chemicals in the body that cause inflammation and pain.

Acetaminophen is generally considered safe to use during pregnancy when taken as directed. However, as with any medication, it is important for pregnant women to speak with their healthcare provider before taking acetaminophen or any other medication during pregnancy. The American College of Obstetricians and Gynecologists (ACOG) recommends that pregnant women use acetaminophen for pain relief instead of nonsteroidal anti-inflammatory drugs (NSAIDs) like ibuprofen and naproxen, as these medications may increase the risk of bleeding and complications during pregnancy.

It is important to follow the recommended dosage and frequency for acetaminophen, as taking too much acetaminophen can cause liver damage. The maximum daily dose of acetaminophen for pregnant women is generally considered to be 4,000 milligrams (mg) per day. However, it is always best to consult with a healthcare provider or pharmacist before taking any medication during pregnancy.

In addition to pain relief, acetaminophen may also be used to reduce fever during pregnancy. It is important to keep in mind that fever during pregnancy can be a sign of an underlying infection, and it is important to speak with a healthcare provider if a fever persists or is accompanied by other symptoms.

Acetaminophen is also available in combination with other medications, such as decongestants, antihistamines, and cough suppressants. It is important to read the label and be aware of all the ingredients in a medication before taking it during pregnancy.

It is also important to be aware of potential drug interactions when taking acetaminophen during pregnancy. Acetaminophen may interact with certain medications, such as blood thinners, anti-depressants, and other pain medications. It is important to speak with a healthcare provider or pharmacist about any medications that are being taken before taking acetaminophen.

Overall, acetaminophen is a safe and effective option for pain relief and fever reduction during pregnancy when taken as directed. However, it is important for pregnant women to speak with their healthcare provider before taking any medication during pregnancy and to follow the recommended dosage and frequency. It is always best to consult with a healthcare provider or pharmacist before taking any medication during pregnancy.

Alcohol

Alcohol is a substance that is found in a wide range of beverages, including beer, wine, and spirits. It is produced by the fermentation of sugars and is commonly consumed for its psychoactive effects.

The consumption of alcohol during pregnancy can be harmful to the developing fetus and is generally not recommended. Alcohol can pass from the mother's blood into the baby's blood, and high levels of alcohol in the baby's blood can cause abnormal fetal development and result in a range of birth defects, known as fetal alcohol spectrum disorders (FASDs).

The effects of alcohol on the developing fetus can be severe and long-lasting, and can include physical abnormalities, brain damage, and developmental delays. There is no known safe amount of alcohol that can be consumed during pregnancy, and no safe time during pregnancy to drink alcohol.

The Centers for Disease Control and Prevention (CDC) recommends that pregnant women abstain from alcohol completely during pregnancy to reduce the risk of FASDs. The CDC also recommends that women who are planning to become pregnant should abstain from alcohol to reduce the risk of unintended pregnancy and the potential harm to the developing fetus.

It is important for pregnant women who are struggling with alcohol use disorder to seek help and support to quit drinking. There are many resources available to help pregnant women who are struggling with alcohol use, including support groups, therapy, and medications.

Overall, the consumption of alcohol during pregnancy can have serious and long-lasting consequences for the developing fetus. It is important for pregnant women to abstain from alcohol to reduce the risk of FASDs and other negative outcomes for the baby.

Almond butter

Almond butter is a type of nut butter made from ground almonds. It is similar to peanut butter and can be used as a spread or an ingredient in a variety of dishes. Almond butter is a good source of protein, fiber, and nutrients such as vitamin E, magnesium, and zinc.

Almond butter is generally considered safe to consume during pregnancy in moderation. Eating a variety of nuts, including almonds, during pregnancy can provide important nutrients and contribute to a healthy diet. However, it is important for pregnant women to be mindful of their intake of nuts, as they are high in calories and should be consumed in moderation as part of an overall balanced diet.

It is also important for pregnant women with allergies or sensitivities to nuts to avoid consuming almond butter and other nut butters. Allergic reactions to nuts can range from mild to severe and can include symptoms such as hives, difficulty breathing, and anaphylaxis. Pregnant women with allergies or sensitivities to nuts should speak with their healthcare provider about the best options for managing their allergy during pregnancy.

In addition, pregnant women should be aware of the risk of contracting listeriosis, a bacterial infection that can be caused by consuming contaminated food. Nuts, including almonds, can be a source of listeriosis if they are contaminated with the bacterium Listeria monocytogenes. Pregnant women are at an increased risk of contracting listeriosis and experiencing severe illness as a result. To reduce the risk of listeriosis, pregnant women should thoroughly wash and properly store nuts, and should avoid consuming nuts that are past their expiration date or have an off smell or taste.

Overall, almond butter can be a nutritious and enjoyable part of a healthy diet during pregnancy when consumed in moderation and with appropriate precautions. As with any food, it is important for pregnant women to speak with their healthcare provider about their dietary needs and any potential risks or concerns.

Almonds

Almonds are a type of tree nut that are often consumed as a snack or used as an ingredient in a variety of dishes. They are a good source of protein, fiber, and nutrients such as vitamin E, magnesium, and zinc. Almonds are generally considered safe to consume during pregnancy in moderation.

Eating a variety of nuts, including almonds, during pregnancy can provide important nutrients and contribute to a healthy diet. However, it is important for pregnant women to be mindful of their intake of nuts, as they are high in calories and should be consumed in moderation as part of an overall balanced diet.

It is also important for pregnant women with allergies or sensitivities to nuts to avoid consuming almonds and other nuts. Allergic reactions to nuts can range from mild to severe and can include symptoms such as hives, difficulty breathing, and anaphylaxis. Pregnant women with allergies or sensitivities to nuts should speak with their healthcare provider about the best options for managing their allergy during pregnancy.

In addition, pregnant women should be aware of the risk of contracting listeriosis, a bacterial infection that can be caused by consuming contaminated food. Nuts, including almonds, can be a source of listeriosis if they are contaminated with the bacterium Listeria monocytogenes. Pregnant women are at an increased risk of contracting listeriosis and experiencing severe illness as a result. To reduce the risk of listeriosis, pregnant women should thoroughly wash and properly store nuts, and should avoid consuming nuts that are past their expiration date or have an off smell or taste.

Overall, almonds can be a nutritious and enjoyable part of a healthy diet during pregnancy when consumed in moderation and with appropriate precautions. As with any food, it is important for pregnant women to speak with their healthcare provider about their dietary needs and any potential risks or concerns.

Applesauce

Applesauce is generally considered safe to eat during pregnancy. It is a good source of several essential nutrients, including vitamin C, potassium, and fiber, which are important for fetal development and the health of the mother.

However, it is important to choose unsweetened applesauce during pregnancy to help control sugar intake and reduce the risk of gestational diabetes and other pregnancy complications. It is also a good idea to avoid consuming large amounts of applesauce or other high-sugar foods if you are prone to developing gestational diabetes, as these foods can contribute to weight gain and increase the risk of developing this condition.

In addition, it is important to follow proper food safety guidelines when consuming applesauce or any other food during pregnancy. This includes checking the expiration date and discarding any applesauce that is spoiled or shows signs of spoilage.

Overall, applesauce can be a healthy and nutritious addition to the diet of a pregnant woman, as long as it is consumed in moderation and as part of a balanced diet. It is a good idea to consult with a healthcare provider or a registered dietitian for personalized nutrition advice.

Aromatherapy

Aromatherapy is a type of complementary and alternative medicine that involves the use of essential oils extracted from plants for their therapeutic properties. Aromatherapy is often used to promote relaxation, improve mood, and reduce stress and anxiety.

There is limited research on the safety and effectiveness of aromatherapy during pregnancy, and the use of essential oils during pregnancy should be approached with caution. Some essential oils, such as clary sage, basil, and fennel, may stimulate contractions and should be avoided during pregnancy. Other essential oils, such as peppermint, may cause heartburn and should be used with caution during pregnancy.

It is important for pregnant women to speak with their healthcare provider before using essential oils or any other complementary or alternative therapy during pregnancy. Pregnant women should also be aware that some essential oils may not be safe to use during pregnancy or may need to be used with caution, as they may be absorbed through the skin and pass into the bloodstream.

Overall, the use of essential oils and aromatherapy during pregnancy should be approached with caution, and pregnant women should speak with their healthcare provider before using these therapies.

Artichokes

Artichokes are a type of vegetable with a characteristic, spiky appearance. They are a good source of fiber, vitamins, and minerals, including vitamin C, potassium, and magnesium. Artichokes are generally considered safe to consume during pregnancy when prepared and consumed properly.

Eating a variety of vegetables, including artichokes, during pregnancy can provide important nutrients and contribute to a healthy diet. However, it is important for pregnant women to be mindful of the risk of contracting foodborne illness, as they are at an increased risk of severe illness as a result of certain types of infections.

To reduce the risk of foodborne illness, pregnant women should thoroughly wash and properly store fresh produce, and should avoid consuming produce that is past its expiration date or has an off smell or taste. Pregnant women should also be careful to fully cook artichokes and other vegetables to kill any harmful bacteria that may be present.

In addition, pregnant women should be aware of the risk of contracting listeriosis, a bacterial infection that can be caused by consuming contaminated food. Artichokes and other vegetables can be a source of listeriosis if they are contaminated with the bacterium Listeria monocytogenes. Pregnant women are at an increased risk of contracting listeriosis and experiencing severe illness as a result. To reduce the risk of listeriosis, pregnant women should thoroughly wash and properly store vegetables, and should avoid consuming vegetables that are past their expiration date or have an off smell or taste.

Overall, artichokes can be a nutritious and enjoyable part of a healthy diet.

Artificial additives and preservatives

Artificial additives and preservatives are substances that are added to food to enhance its taste, appearance, or shelf life. Examples of artificial additives and preservatives include food coloring, flavorings, and preservatives such as sodium benzoate and sodium nitrite.

The safety of artificial additives and preservatives during pregnancy is a controversial topic and the subject of ongoing research. Some studies have suggested that certain artificial additives and preservatives may be harmful to pregnant women and their developing fetuses, while others have found no negative effects.

The Food and Drug Administration (FDA) has set safe limits for the use of artificial additives and preservatives in food. However, it is important for pregnant women to be aware that the safety of these substances during pregnancy has not been fully established, and to use caution when consuming foods that contain artificial additives and preservatives.

Pregnant women who are concerned about the potential effects of artificial additives and preservatives on their health and the health of their developing fetus may choose to limit their consumption of processed and packaged foods, which are more likely to contain these substances. Instead, they may opt for whole, unprocessed foods, which are generally considered to be healthier options.

Overall, it is important for pregnant women to be mindful of their intake of artificial additives and preservatives, and to speak with their healthcare provider about any concerns they may have.

Artificial sweeteners

Artificial sweeteners are substances that are used to sweeten foods and beverages without adding calories or increasing blood sugar levels. Some examples of artificial sweeteners include aspartame, sucralose, and stevia.

The safety of artificial sweeteners during pregnancy is a controversial topic and the subject of ongoing research. Some studies have suggested that certain artificial sweeteners may be harmful to pregnant women and their developing fetuses, while others have found no negative effects.

The Food and Drug Administration (FDA) has approved several artificial sweeteners for use in food, including aspartame, sucralose, and stevia. However, it is important for pregnant women to be aware that the safety of these substances during pregnancy has not been fully established, and to use caution when consuming foods and beverages that contain artificial sweeteners.

Pregnant women who are concerned about the potential effects of artificial sweeteners on their health and the health of their developing fetus may choose to limit their consumption of foods and beverages that contain these substances. Instead, they may opt for natural sweeteners, such as honey or maple syrup, or may choose to reduce their overall intake of sweetened foods and beverages.

It is important for pregnant women to speak with their healthcare provider about their dietary needs and any concerns they may have about the use of artificial sweeteners during pregnancy.

Asparagus

Asparagus is a type of vegetable with a long, thin, green stalk. It is a good source of fiber, vitamins, and minerals, including vitamin K, vitamin C, and potassium. Asparagus is generally considered safe to consume during pregnancy when prepared and consumed properly.

Eating a variety of vegetables, including asparagus, during pregnancy can provide important nutrients and contribute to a healthy diet. However, it is important for pregnant women to be mindful of the risk of contracting foodborne illness, as they are at an increased risk of severe illness as a result of certain types of infections.

To reduce the risk of foodborne illness, pregnant women should thoroughly wash and properly store fresh produce, and should avoid consuming produce that is past its expiration date or has an off smell or taste. Pregnant women should also be careful to fully cook asparagus and other vegetables to kill any harmful bacteria that may be present.

In addition, pregnant women should be aware of the risk of contracting listeriosis, a bacterial infection that can be caused by consuming contaminated food. Asparagus and other vegetables can be a source of listeriosis if they are contaminated with the bacterium Listeria monocytogenes. Pregnant women are at an increased risk of contracting listeriosis and experiencing severe illness as a result. To reduce the risk of listeriosis, pregnant women should thoroughly wash and properly store vegetables, and should avoid consuming vegetables that are past their expiration date or have an off smell or taste.

Overall, asparagus can be a nutritious and enjoyable part of a healthy diet during pregnancy when consumed in moderation and with appropriate precautions. As with any food, it is important for pregnant women to speak with their healthcare provider about their dietary needs and any potential risks or concerns.

Avocado

Avocado is a type of fruit with a creamy, green flesh and a large, inedible seed. It is a good source of healthy fats, fiber, and nutrients, such as potassium, vitamin E, and folate. Avocado is generally considered safe to consume during pregnancy when prepared and consumed properly.

Eating a variety of fruits, including avocado, during pregnancy can provide important nutrients and contribute to a healthy diet. However, it is important for pregnant women to be mindful of the risk of contracting foodborne illness, as they are at an increased risk of severe illness as a result of certain types of infections.

To reduce the risk of foodborne illness, pregnant women should thoroughly wash and properly store fresh produce, and should avoid consuming produce that is past its expiration date or has an off smell or taste. Pregnant women should also be careful to fully cook avocado and other fruits to kill any harmful bacteria that may be present.

In addition, pregnant women should be aware of the risk of contracting listeriosis, a bacterial infection that can be caused by consuming contaminated food. Avocado and other fruits can be a source of listeriosis if they are contaminated with the bacterium Listeria monocytogenes. Pregnant women are at an increased risk of contracting listeriosis and experiencing severe illness as a result. To reduce the risk of listeriosis, pregnant women should thoroughly wash and properly store fruits, and should avoid consuming fruits that are past their expiration date or have an off smell or taste.

Overall, avocado can be a nutritious and enjoyable part of a healthy diet during pregnancy when consumed in moderation and with appropriate precautions. As with any food, it is important for pregnant women to speak with their healthcare provider about their dietary needs and any potential risks or concerns.

Ayurvedic medicine

Ayurvedic medicine is a system of traditional medicine that originated in India and has been practiced for thousands of years. It is based on the belief that health and wellness depend on a balance between the body, mind, and spirit. Ayurvedic medicine uses a variety of techniques, including herbal remedies, diet, and lifestyle changes, to treat a range of conditions and maintain overall health.

There is limited research on the safety and effectiveness of Ayurvedic medicine during pregnancy, and the use of Ayurvedic remedies during pregnancy should be approached with caution. Some herbs and other substances used in Ayurvedic medicine may not be safe to use during pregnancy or may need to be used with caution, as they may be absorbed through the skin and pass into the bloodstream.

It is important for pregnant women to speak with their healthcare provider before using Ayurvedic remedies or any other complementary or alternative therapy during pregnancy. Pregnant women should also be aware that some Ayurvedic remedies may not be regulated by the Food and Drug Administration (FDA) and may contain undisclosed ingredients or contaminants.

Overall, the use of Ayurvedic medicine during pregnancy should be approached with caution, and pregnant women should speak with their healthcare provider before using these therapies.

Baby carrots

Baby carrots are generally considered safe to eat during pregnancy. They are a good source of several essential nutrients, including vitamin A, vitamin C, potassium, and fiber, which are important for fetal development and the health of the mother.

However, it is important to follow proper food safety guidelines when consuming baby carrots or any other produce during pregnancy. This includes washing the carrots thoroughly to remove any dirt or contaminants, and discarding any carrots that are spoiled or show signs of spoilage.

In addition, it is recommended to avoid consuming large amounts of baby carrots or other high-fiber foods if you have a history of kidney stones, as these foods are high in oxalates and may increase the risk of developing kidney stones.

Overall, baby carrots can be a healthy and nutritious addition to the diet of a pregnant woman, as long as they are properly prepared and consumed in moderation as part of a balanced diet. It is a good idea to consult with a healthcare provider or a registered dietitian for personalized nutrition advice.

Baked potatoes

Baked potatoes are generally considered safe to eat during pregnancy. They are a good source of several essential nutrients, including potassium, vitamin C, and fiber, which are important for fetal development and the health of the mother.

However, it is important to choose baked potatoes that are prepared in a healthy way, such as by baking or microwaving, rather than deep-frying or loading them with unhealthy toppings like cheese, bacon, and sour cream. These toppings can add unhealthy amounts of salt, saturated fat, and calories to the potato and increase the risk of gestational diabetes and other pregnancy complications.

In addition, it is important to follow proper food safety guidelines when consuming baked potatoes or any other food during pregnancy. This includes checking the expiration date and discarding any potatoes that are spoiled or show signs of spoilage.

Overall, baked potatoes can be a healthy and nutritious addition to the diet of a pregnant woman, as long as they are prepared in a healthy way and consumed in moderation as part of a balanced diet. It is a good idea to consult with a healthcare provider or a registered dietitian for personalized nutrition advice.

Banana bread

Banana bread is a type of baked goods that is made with mashed bananas and flour as the main ingredients. While it can be a tasty and convenient snack option, it is important to choose banana bread that is nutritious and safe to eat during pregnancy.

Many store-bought and homemade banana breads are high in added sugars, salt, and unhealthy fats, and provide little nutritional value. These types of banana breads can contribute to weight gain and increase the risk of gestational diabetes and other pregnancy complications.

It is a good idea to choose banana bread that is made with whole grain flour and natural sweeteners, such as honey or maple syrup, and to limit the intake of added sugars and unhealthy fats. You can also make your own banana bread at home using healthier ingredients, such as whole grain flour, ripe bananas, and unsweetened applesauce or coconut oil, to control the nutritional content of the bread.

In addition, it is important to follow proper food safety guidelines when consuming banana bread or any other food during pregnancy. This includes checking the expiration date and discarding any banana bread that is spoiled or shows signs of spoilage.

Overall, it is a good idea to choose banana bread that is nutritious and safe to eat during pregnancy, and to consume it in moderation as part of a balanced diet. It is a good idea to consult with a healthcare provider or a registered dietitian for personalized nutrition advice.

Bananas

Bananas are a type of fruit with a yellow, peeled skin and a soft, creamy flesh. They are a good source of potassium, vitamin C, and fiber. Bananas are generally considered safe to consume during pregnancy when prepared and consumed properly.

Eating a variety of fruits, including bananas, during pregnancy can provide important nutrients and contribute to a healthy diet. However, it is important for pregnant women to be mindful of the risk of contracting foodborne illness, as they are at an increased risk of severe illness as a result of certain types of infections.

To reduce the risk of foodborne illness, pregnant women should thoroughly wash and properly store fresh produce, and should avoid consuming produce that is past its expiration date or has an off smell or taste. Pregnant women should also be careful to fully cook bananas and other fruits to kill any harmful bacteria that may be present.

In addition, pregnant women should be aware of the risk of contracting listeriosis, a bacterial infection that can be caused by consuming contaminated food. Bananas and other fruits can be a source of listeriosis if they are contaminated with the bacterium Listeria monocytogenes. Pregnant women are at an increased risk of contracting listeriosis and experiencing severe illness as a result. To reduce the risk of listeriosis, pregnant lunt women should thoroughly wash and properly store fruits, and should avoid consuming fruits that are past their expiration date or have an off smell or taste.

Overall, bananas can be a nutritious and enjoyable part of a healthy diet during pregnancy when consumed in moderation and with appropriate precautions. As with any food, it is important for pregnant women to speak with their healthcare provider about their dietary needs and any potential risks or concerns.

BBQ sauce

BBQ sauce is a condiment that is used to flavor grilled or roasted meats and vegetables. While it can be a tasty addition to many dishes, it is important to choose BBQ sauce that is nutritious and safe to eat during pregnancy.

Many store-bought and homemade BBQ sauces are high in added sugars, salt, and unhealthy fats, and provide little nutritional value. These types of BBQ sauces can contribute to weight gain and increase the risk of gestational diabetes and other pregnancy complications.

It is a good idea to choose BBQ sauces that are made with healthier ingredients, such as tomato paste, vinegar, and natural sweeteners, and to limit the intake of added sugars and unhealthy fats. You can also make your own BBQ sauce at home using healthier ingredients, such as tomato paste, vinegar, honey, and spices, to control the nutritional content of the sauce.

In addition, it is important to follow proper food safety guidelines when consuming BBQ sauce or any other food during pregnancy. This includes checking the expiration date and discarding any BBQ sauce that is spoiled or shows signs of spoilage.

Overall, it is a good idea to choose BBQ sauce that is nutritious and safe to eat during pregnancy, and to consume it in moderation as part of a balanced diet. It is a good idea to consult with a healthcare provider or a registered dietitian for personalized nutrition advice.

Beans

Beans are a type of legume with a hard outer shell and a soft, edible interior. They are a good source of protein, fiber, and nutrients, such as iron, potassium, and folate. Beans are generally considered safe to consume during pregnancy when prepared and consumed properly.

Eating a variety of protein-rich foods, including beans, during pregnancy can provide important nutrients and contribute to a healthy diet. However, it is important for pregnant women to be mindful of the risk of contracting foodborne illness, as they are at an increased risk of severe illness as a result of certain types of infections.

To reduce the risk of foodborne illness, pregnant women should thoroughly wash and properly store fresh produce, and should avoid consuming produce that is past its expiration date or has an off smell or taste. Pregnant women should also be careful to fully cook beans and other legumes to kill any harmful bacteria that may be present.

In addition, pregnant women should be aware of the risk of contracting listeriosis, a bacterial infection that can be caused by consuming contaminated food. Beans and other legumes can be a source of listeriosis if they are contaminated with the bacterium Listeria monocytogenes. Pregnant women are at an increased risk of contracting listeriosis and experiencing severe illness as a result. To reduce the risk of listeriosis, pregnant women should thoroughly wash and properly store legumes, and should avoid consuming legumes that are past their expiration date or have an off smell or taste.

Overall, beans can be a nutritious and enjoyable part of a healthy diet during pregnancy when consumed in moderation and with appropriate precautions. As with any food, it is important for pregnant women to speak with their healthcare provider about their dietary needs and any potential risks or concerns.

Beef jerky

Beef jerky is a type of snack food that is made by drying slices of beef until they are chewy and then seasoning them with various spices and flavors. While it can be a convenient and tasty snack option, it is important to choose beef jerky that is nutritious and safe to eat during pregnancy.

Many store-bought and homemade beef jerky products are high in salt, added sugars, and unhealthy fats, and provide little nutritional value. These types of beef jerky can contribute to weight gain and increase the risk of gestational diabetes and other pregnancy complications.

It is a good idea to choose beef jerky that is made with healthier ingredients, such as lean cuts of beef, natural sweeteners, and minimal amounts of salt and unhealthy fats, and to limit the intake of added sugars and unhealthy fats. You can also make your own beef jerky at home using healthier ingredients, such as lean cuts of beef, natural sweeteners, and spices, to control the nutritional content of the jerky.

In addition, it is important to follow proper food safety guidelines when consuming beef jerky or any other food during pregnancy. This includes checking the expiration date and discarding any beef jerky that is spoiled or shows signs of spoilage.

Overall, it is a good idea to choose beef jerky that is nutritious and safe to eat during pregnancy, and to consume it in moderation as part of a balanced diet. It is a good idea to consult with a healthcare provider or a registered dietitian for personalized nutrition advice.

Beet greens

Beet greens are the edible leaves of the beet plant. They are a good source of vitamins, minerals, and fiber. Beet greens are generally considered safe to consume during pregnancy when prepared and consumed properly.

Eating a variety of vegetables, including beet greens, during pregnancy can provide important nutrients and contribute to a healthy diet. However, it is important for pregnant women to be mindful of the risk of contracting foodborne illness, as they are at an increased risk of severe illness as a result of certain types of infections.

To reduce the risk of foodborne illness, pregnant women should thoroughly wash and properly store fresh produce, and should avoid consuming produce that is past its expiration date or has an off smell or taste. Pregnant women should also be careful to fully cook beet greens and other vegetables to kill any harmful bacteria that may be present.

In addition, pregnant women should be aware of the risk of contracting listeriosis, a bacterial infection that can be caused by consuming contaminated food. Beet greens and other vegetables can be a source of listeriosis if they are contaminated with the bacterium Listeria monocytogenes. Pregnant women are at an increased risk of contracting listeriosis and experiencing severe illness as a result. To reduce the risk of listeriosis, pregnant women should thoroughly wash and properly store vegetables, and should avoid consuming vegetables that are past their expiration date or have an off smell or taste.

Overall, beet greens can be a nutritious and enjoyable part of a healthy diet during pregnancy when consumed in moderation and with appropriate precautions. As with any food, it is important for pregnant women to speak with their healthcare provider about their dietary needs and any potential risks or concerns.

Beets

Beets are a type of vegetable with a red or purple flesh and a sweet, earthy flavor. They are a good source of vitamins, minerals, and fiber. Beets are generally considered safe to consume during pregnancy when prepared and consumed properly.

Eating a variety of vegetables, including beets, during pregnancy can provide important nutrients and contribute to a healthy diet. However, it is important for pregnant women to be mindful of the risk of contracting foodborne illness, as they are at an increased risk of severe illness as a result of certain types of infections.

To reduce the risk of foodborne illness, pregnant women should thoroughly wash and properly store fresh produce, and should avoid consuming produce that is past its expiration date or has an off smell or taste. Pregnant women should also be careful to fully cook beets and other vegetables to kill any harmful bacteria that may be present.

In addition, pregnant women should be aware of the risk of contracting listeriosis, a bacterial infection that can be caused by consuming contaminated food. Beets and other vegetables can be a source of listeriosis if they are contaminated with the bacterium Listeria monocytogenes. Pregnant women are at an increased risk of contracting listeriosis and experiencing severe illness as a result. To reduce the risk of listeriosis, pregnant women should thoroughly wash and properly store vegetables, and should avoid consuming vegetables that are past their expiration date or have an off smell or taste.

Overall, beets can be a nutritious and enjoyable part of a healthy diet during pregnancy when consumed in moderation and with appropriate precautions. As with any food, it is important for pregnant women to speak with their healthcare provider about their dietary needs and any potential risks or concerns.

Berries such as strawberries, raspberries, and blueberries

Berries, including strawberries, raspberries, and blueberries, are small, sweet fruits that are a good source of vitamins, minerals, and fiber. Berries are generally considered safe to consume during pregnancy when prepared and consumed properly.

Eating a variety of fruits, including berries, during pregnancy can provide important nutrients and contribute to a healthy diet. However, it is important for pregnant women to be mindful of the risk of contracting foodborne illness, as they are at an increased risk of severe illness as a result of certain types of infections.

To reduce the risk of foodborne illness, pregnant women should thoroughly wash and properly store fresh produce, and should avoid consuming produce that is past its expiration date or has an off smell or taste. Pregnant women should also be careful to fully cook berries and other fruits to kill any harmful bacteria that may be present.

In addition, pregnant women should be aware of the risk of contracting listeriosis, a bacterial infection that can be caused by consuming contaminated food. Berries and other fruits can be a source of listeriosis if they are contaminated with the bacterium Listeria monocytogenes. Pregnant women are at an increased risk of contracting listeriosis and experiencing severe illness as a result. To reduce the risk of listeriosis, pregnant women should thoroughly wash and properly store fruits, and should avoid consuming fruits that are past their expiration date or have an off smell or taste.

Overall, berries can be a nutritious and enjoyable part of a healthy diet during pregnancy when consumed in moderation and with appropriate precautions. As with any food, it is important for pregnant women to speak with their healthcare provider about their dietary needs and any potential risks or concerns.

Black beans

Black beans are a type of legume with a hard outer shell and a soft, edible interior. They are a good source of protein, fiber, and nutrients, such as iron, potassium, and folate. Black beans are generally considered safe to consume during pregnancy when prepared and consumed properly.

Eating a variety of protein-rich foods, including black beans, during pregnancy can provide important nutrients and contribute to a healthy diet. However, it is important for pregnant women to be mindful of the risk of contracting foodborne illness, as they are at an increased risk of severe illness as a result of certain types of infections.

To reduce the risk of foodborne illness, pregnant women should thoroughly wash and properly store fresh produce, and should avoid consuming produce that is past its expiration date or has an off smell or taste. Pregnant women should also be careful to fully cook black beans and other legumes to kill any harmful bacteria that may be present.

In addition, pregnant women should be aware of the risk of contracting listeriosis, a bacterial infection that can be caused by consuming contaminated food. Black beans and other legumes can be a source of listeriosis if they are contaminated with the bacterium Listeria monocytogenes. Pregnant women are at an increased risk of contracting listeriosis and experiencing severe illness as a result. To reduce the risk of listeriosis, pregnant women should thoroughly wash and properly store legumes, and should avoid consuming legumes that are past their expiration date or have an off smell or taste.

Overall, black beans can be a nutritious and enjoyable part of a healthy diet during pregnancy when consumed in moderation and with appropriate precautions. As with any food, it is important for pregnant women to speak with their healthcare provider about their dietary needs and any potential risks or concerns.

Blue cheese dressing

Blue cheese dressing is a type of salad dressing that is made with blue cheese, milk, and other ingredients. While it can be a tasty addition to many dishes, it is important to choose blue cheese dressing that is nutritious and safe to eat during pregnancy.

Blue cheese is made from cow's milk and is a source of protein, calcium, and other nutrients. However, it is also high in salt and saturated fat, and consuming large amounts of these nutrients can increase the risk of gestational diabetes and other pregnancy complications.

In addition, it is important to follow proper food safety guidelines when consuming blue cheese dressing or any other food during pregnancy. This includes checking the expiration date and discarding any blue cheese dressing that is spoiled or shows signs of spoilage.

It is a good idea to choose blue cheese dressing that is made with healthier ingredients, such as low-fat milk and minimal amounts of salt and unhealthy fats, and to limit the intake of added sugars and unhealthy fats. You can also make your own blue cheese dressing at home using healthier ingredients, such as low-fat milk, blue cheese, and spices, to control the nutritional content of the dressing.

Overall, it is a good idea to choose blue cheese dressing that is nutritious and safe to eat during pregnancy, and to consume it in moderation as part of a balanced diet. It is a good idea to consult with a healthcare provider or a registered dietitian for personalized nutrition advice.

Blueberries

Blueberries are a type of small, sweet fruit with a blue or purple skin and a soft, edible interior. They are a good source of vitamins, minerals, and fiber. Blueberries are generally considered safe to consume during pregnancy when prepared and consumed properly.

Eating a variety of fruits, including blueberries, during pregnancy can provide important nutrients and contribute to a healthy diet. However, it is important for pregnant women to be mindful of the risk of contracting foodborne illness, as they are at an increased risk of severe illness as a result of certain types of infections.

To reduce the risk of foodborne illness, pregnant women should thoroughly wash and properly store fresh produce, and should avoid consuming produce that is past its expiration date or has an off smell or taste. Pregnant women should also be careful to fully cook blueberries and other fruits to kill any harmful bacteria that may be present.

In addition, pregnant women should be aware of the risk of contracting listeriosis, a bacterial infection that can be caused by consuming contaminated food. Blueberries and other fruits can be a source of listeriosis if they are contaminated with the bacterium Listeria monocytogenes. Pregnant women are at an increased risk of contracting listeriosis and experiencing severe illness as a result. To reduce the risk of listeriosis, pregnant women should thoroughly wash and properly store fruits, and should avoid consuming fruits that are past their expiration date or have an off smell or taste.

Overall, blueberries can be a nutritious and enjoyable part of a healthy diet during pregnancy when consumed in moderation and with appropriate precautions. As with any food, it is important for pregnant women to speak with their healthcare provider about their dietary needs and any potential risks or concerns.

Bran flakes

Bran flakes are a type of breakfast cereal made from wheat bran, which is the outer layer of the wheat grain. They are a good source of several essential nutrients, including fiber, protein, and several vitamins and minerals, which are important for fetal development and the health of the mother.

However, it is important to choose bran flakes that are made with whole grain wheat bran, as this type of bran is more nutritious and provides more fiber and other nutrients than refined wheat bran. It is also a good idea to choose bran flakes that are low in added sugars, salt, and unhealthy fats, and to limit the intake of these nutrients during pregnancy.

In addition, it is important to follow proper food safety guidelines when consuming bran flakes or any other food during pregnancy. This includes checking the expiration date and discarding any bran flakes that are spoiled or show signs of spoilage.

Overall, bran flakes can be a healthy and nutritious addition to the diet of a pregnant woman, as long as they are made with whole grain wheat bran and consumed in moderation as part of a balanced diet. It is a good idea to consult with a healthcare provider or a registered dietitian for personalized nutrition advice.

Breadcrumbs

Bread crumbs are small, dry pieces of bread that are used as a filler or coating in various dishes. While they can be a convenient and tasty ingredient, it is important to choose bread crumbs that are nutritious and safe to eat during pregnancy.

Many store-bought and homemade bread crumbs are made with refined grains, which are lower in nutrients and fiber than whole grains. It is a good idea to choose bread crumbs that are made with whole grain bread, as this type of bread is more nutritious and provides more fiber and other nutrients than refined grain bread.

In addition, it is important to follow proper food safety guidelines when consuming bread crumbs or any other food during pregnancy. This includes checking the expiration date and discarding any bread crumbs that are spoiled or show signs of spoilage.

Overall, bread crumbs can be a healthy and nutritious addition to the diet of a pregnant woman, as long as they are made with whole grain bread and consumed in moderation as part of a balanced diet. It is a good idea to consult with a healthcare provider or a registered dietitian for personalized nutrition advice.

Breaded chicken

Breaded chicken is a type of chicken that is coated with bread crumbs or other types of flour and then fried or baked. While it can be a tasty and convenient snack or meal option, it is important to choose breaded chicken that is nutritious and safe to eat during pregnancy.

Many store-bought and homemade breaded chicken products are high in salt, added sugars, and unhealthy fats, and provide little nutritional value. These types of breaded chicken can contribute to weight gain and increase the risk of gestational diabetes and other pregnancy complications.

It is a good idea to choose breaded chicken that is made with healthier ingredients, such as whole grain flour and minimal amounts of salt and unhealthy fats, and to limit the intake of added sugars and unhealthy fats. You can also make your own breaded chicken at home using healthier ingredients, such as whole grain flour, spices, and herbs, to control the nutritional content of the chicken.

In addition, it is important to follow proper food safety guidelines when consuming breaded chicken or any other food during pregnancy. This includes checking the expiration date and discarding any breaded chicken that is spoiled or shows signs of spoilage.

Overall, it is a good idea to choose breaded chicken that is nutritious and safe to eat during pregnancy, and to consume it in moderation as part of a balanced diet. It is a good idea to consult with a healthcare provider or a registered dietitian for personalized nutrition advice.

Broth

Broth is a type of liquid that is made by simmering bones, vegetables, and other ingredients in water. It is often used as a base for soups, stews, and other dishes. While broth can be a tasty and convenient ingredient, it is important to choose broth that is nutritious and safe to eat during pregnancy.

Many store-bought and homemade broths are high in salt, which can contribute to high blood pressure and other pregnancy complications. It is a good idea to choose broth that is low in salt or made with minimal amounts of salt, and to limit the intake of salt during pregnancy.

In addition, it is important to follow proper food safety guidelines when consuming broth or any other food during pregnancy. This includes checking the expiration date and discarding any broth that is spoiled or shows signs of spoilage.

Overall, broth can be a healthy and nutritious addition to the diet of a pregnant woman, as long as it is made with low-salt or minimal amounts of salt and consumed in moderation as part of a balanced diet. It is a good idea to consult with a healthcare provider or a registered dietitian for personalized nutrition advice.

Brownies

Brownies are a type of baked goods that are made with chocolate, sugar, and other ingredients. While they can be a tasty and convenient snack or dessert option, it is important to choose brownies that are nutritious and safe to eat during pregnancy.

Many store-bought and homemade brownies are high in added sugars, salt, and unhealthy fats, and provide little nutritional value. These types of brownies can contribute to weight gain and increase the risk of gestational diabetes and other pregnancy complications.

It is a good idea to choose brownies that are made with healthier ingredients, such as whole grain flour, natural sweeteners, and minimal amounts of salt and unhealthy fats, and to limit the intake of added sugars and unhealthy fats. You can also make your own brownies at home using healthier ingredients, such as whole grain flour, cocoa powder, natural sweeteners, and unsweetened applesauce or coconut oil, to control the nutritional content of the brownies.

In addition, it is important to follow proper food safety guidelines when consuming brownies or any other food during pregnancy. This includes checking the expiration date and discarding any brownies that are spoiled or show signs of spoilage.

Overall, it is a good idea to choose brownies that are nutritious and safe to eat during pregnancy, and to consume them in moderation as part of a balanced diet. It is a good idea to consult with a healthcare provider or a registered dietitian for personalized nutrition advice.

Buffalo sauce

Buffalo sauce is a spicy condiment that is made with hot sauce, vinegar, and other ingredients. While it can be a tasty addition to many dishes, it is important to choose buffalo sauce that is nutritious and safe to eat during pregnancy.

Many store-bought and homemade buffalo sauces are high in salt, added sugars, and unhealthy fats, and provide little nutritional value. These types of buffalo sauces can contribute to weight gain and increase the risk of gestational diabetes and other pregnancy complications.

It is a good idea to choose buffalo sauces that are made with healthier ingredients, such as hot sauce, vinegar, and minimal amounts of salt and unhealthy fats, and to limit the intake of added sugars and unhealthy fats. You can also make your own buffalo sauce at home using healthier ingredients, such as hot sauce, vinegar, and spices, to control the nutritional content of the sauce.

In addition, it is important to follow proper food safety guidelines when consuming buffalo sauce or any other food during pregnancy. This includes checking the expiration date and discarding any buffalo sauce that is spoiled or shows signs of spoilage.

Overall, it is a good idea to choose buffalo sauce that is nutritious and safe to eat during pregnancy, and to consume it in moderation as part of a balanced diet. It is a good idea to consult with a healthcare provider or a registered dietitian for personalized nutrition advice.

Cabbage

Cabbage is a type of leafy vegetable with a crunchy, crisp texture and a slightly sweet, savory flavor. It is a good source of vitamins, minerals, and fiber. Cabbage is generally considered safe to consume during pregnancy when prepared and consumed properly.

Eating a variety of vegetables, including cabbage, during pregnancy can provide important nutrients and contribute to a healthy diet. However, it is important for pregnant women to be mindful of the risk of contracting foodborne illness, as they are at an increased risk of severe illness as a result of certain types of infections.

To reduce the risk of foodborne illness, pregnant women should thoroughly wash and properly store fresh produce, and should avoid consuming produce that is past its expiration date or has an off smell or taste. Pregnant women should also be careful to fully cook cabbage and other vegetables to kill any harmful bacteria that may be present.

In addition, pregnant women should be aware of the risk of contracting listeriosis, a bacterial infection that can be caused by consuming contaminated food. Cabbage and other vegetables can be a source of listeriosis if they are contaminated with the bacterium Listeria monocytogenes. Pregnant women are at an increased risk of contracting listeriosis and experiencing severe illness as a result. To reduce the risk of listeriosis, pregnant women should thoroughly wash and properly store vegetables, and should avoid consuming vegetables that are past their expiration date or have an off smell or taste.

Overall, cabbage can be a nutritious and enjoyable part of a healthy diet during pregnancy when consumed in moderation and with appropriate precautions. As with any food, it is important for pregnant women to speak with their healthcare provider about their dietary needs and any potential risks or concerns.

Cabbage rolls

Cabbage rolls are a type of dish that is made by wrapping ground meat and other fillings in cabbage leaves and then baking or steaming them. While they can be a tasty and nutritious meal option, it is important to choose cabbage rolls that are safe to eat during pregnancy.

It is a good idea to choose cabbage rolls that are made with healthy ingredients, such as lean cuts of meat, whole grains, and vegetables, and to limit the intake of added sugars, salt, and unhealthy fats. You can also make your own cabbage rolls at home using healthier ingredients, such as lean cuts of meat, whole grains, and vegetables, to control the nutritional content of the rolls.

In addition, it is important to follow proper food safety guidelines when consuming cabbage rolls or any other food during pregnancy. This includes washing the ingredients thoroughly to remove any dirt or contaminants, and discarding any cabbage rolls that are spoiled or show signs of spoilage.

Overall, cabbage rolls can be a healthy and nutritious addition to the diet of a pregnant woman, as long as they are made with healthy ingredients and consumed in moderation as part of a balanced diet. It is a good idea to consult with a healthcare provider or a registered dietitian for personalized nutrition advice.

Cajun seasoning

Cajun seasoning is a type of spice blend that is typically made with a combination of paprika, garlic, onion, and other spices. While it can be a tasty and convenient ingredient, it is important to choose Cajun seasoning that is nutritious and safe to eat during pregnancy.

Many store-bought and homemade Cajun seasoning blends are high in salt, which can contribute to high blood pressure and other pregnancy complications. It is a good idea to choose Cajun seasoning that is low in salt or made with minimal amounts of salt, and to limit the intake of salt during pregnancy.

In addition, it is important to follow proper food safety guidelines when consuming Cajun seasoning or any other food during pregnancy. This includes checking the expiration date and discarding any Cajun seasoning that is spoiled or shows signs of spoilage.

Overall, Cajun seasoning can be a healthy and nutritious addition to the diet of a pregnant woman, as long as it is made with low-salt or minimal amounts of salt and consumed in moderation as part of a balanced diet. It is a good idea to consult with a healthcare provider or a registered dietitian for personalized nutrition advice.

Cakes

Cakes are a type of baked goods that are made with flour, sugar, and other ingredients. While they can be a tasty and convenient snack or dessert option, it is important to choose cakes that are nutritious and safe to eat during pregnancy.

Many store-bought and homemade cakes are high in added sugars, salt, and unhealthy fats, and provide little nutritional value. These types of cakes can contribute to weight gain and increase the risk of gestational diabetes and other pregnancy complications.

It is a good idea to choose cakes that are made with healthier ingredients, such as whole grain flour, natural sweeteners, and minimal amounts of salt and unhealthy fats, and to limit the intake of added sugars and unhealthy fats. You can also make your own cakes at home using healthier ingredients, such as whole grain flour, natural sweeteners, and unsweetened applesauce or coconut oil, to control the nutritional content of the cakes.

In addition, it is important to follow proper food safety guidelines when consuming cakes or any other food during pregnancy. This includes checking the expiration date and discarding any cakes that are spoiled or show signs of spoilage.

Overall, it is a good idea to choose cakes that are nutritious and safe to eat during pregnancy, and to consume them in moderation as part of a balanced diet. It is a good idea to consult with a

healthcare provider or a registered dietitian for personalized nutrition advice.

Cantaloupe

Cantaloupe, also known as muskmelon, is a type of fruit that is rich in nutrients, including vitamin C, potassium, and beta-carotene. These nutrients are important for fetal development and the health of the mother during pregnancy.

Cantaloupe is a good source of dietary fiber, which can help to promote healthy digestion and prevent constipation, a common pregnancy complaint. It is also low in calories and fat, making it a healthy and nutritious snack or dessert option for pregnant women.

In addition, it is important to follow proper food safety guidelines when consuming cantaloupe or any other food during pregnancy. This includes washing the fruit thoroughly to remove any dirt or contaminants, and discarding any cantaloupe that is spoiled or shows signs of spoilage.

Overall, cantaloupe can be a healthy and nutritious addition to the diet of a pregnant woman, as long as it is consumed in moderation as part of a balanced diet. It is a good idea to consult with a healthcare provider or a registered dietitian for personalized nutrition advice.

Caramel sauce

Caramel sauce is a sweet, smooth, and thick sauce that is made with caramelized sugar and other ingredients. While it can be a tasty addition to many dishes, it is important to choose caramel sauce that is nutritious and safe to eat during pregnancy.

Many store-bought and homemade caramel sauces are high in added sugars, salt, and unhealthy fats, and provide little nutritional value. These types of caramel sauces can contribute to weight gain and increase the risk of gestational diabetes and other pregnancy complications.

It is a good idea to choose caramel sauces that are made with healthier ingredients, such as natural sweeteners, and minimal amounts of salt and unhealthy fats, and to limit the intake of added sugars and unhealthy fats. You can also make your own caramel sauce at home using healthier ingredients, such as natural sweeteners and unsweetened milk or cream, to control the nutritional content of the sauce.

In addition, it is important to follow proper food safety guidelines when consuming caramel sauce or any other food during pregnancy. This includes checking the expiration date and discarding any caramel sauce that is spoiled or shows signs of spoilage.

Overall, it is a good idea to choose caramel sauce that is nutritious and safe to eat during pregnancy, and to consume it in moderation as part of a balanced diet. It is a good idea to consult with a healthcare provider or a registered dietitian for personalized nutrition advice.

Carrots

Carrots are a type of root vegetable with a sweet, crunchy texture and a bright orange color. They are a good source of vitamins, minerals, and fiber. Carrots are generally considered safe to consume during pregnancy when prepared and consumed properly.

Eating a variety of vegetables, including carrots, during pregnancy can provide important nutrients and contribute to a healthy diet. However, it is important for pregnant women to be mindful of the risk of contracting foodborne illness, as they are at an increased risk of severe illness as a result of certain types of infections.

To reduce the risk of foodborne illness, pregnant women should thoroughly wash and properly store fresh produce, and should avoid consuming produce that is past its expiration date or has an off smell or taste. Pregnant women should also be careful to fully cook carrots and other vegetables to kill any harmful bacteria that may be present.

In addition, pregnant women should be aware of the risk of contracting listeriosis, a bacterial infection that can be caused by consuming contaminated food. Carrots and other vegetables can be a source of listeriosis if they are contaminated with the bacterium Listeria monocytogenes. Pregnant women are at an increased risk of contracting listeriosis and experiencing severe illness as a result. To reduce the risk of listeriosis, pregnant women should thoroughly wash and properly store vegetables, and should avoid consuming vegetables that are past their expiration date or have an off smell or taste.

Overall, carrots can be a nutritious and enjoyable part of a healthy diet during pregnancy when consumed in moderation and with appropriate precautions. As with any food, it is important for pregnant women to speak with their healthcare provider about their dietary needs and any potential risks or concerns.

Cauliflower

Cauliflower is a type of cruciferous vegetable with a mild, slightly sweet flavor and a crunchy, firm texture. It is a good source of vitamins, minerals, and fiber. Cauliflower is generally considered safe to consume during pregnancy when prepared and consumed properly.

Eating a variety of vegetables, including cauliflower, during pregnancy can provide important nutrients and contribute to a healthy diet. However, it is important for pregnant women to be mindful of the risk of contracting foodborne illness, as they are at an increased risk of severe illness as a result of certain types of infections.

To reduce the risk of foodborne illness, pregnant women should thoroughly wash and properly store fresh produce, and should avoid consuming produce that is past its expiration date or has an off smell or taste. Pregnant women should also be careful to fully cook cauliflower and other vegetables to kill any harmful bacteria that may be present.

In addition, pregnant women should be aware of the risk of contracting listeriosis, a bacterial infection that can be caused by consuming contaminated food. Cauliflower and other vegetables can be a source of listeriosis if they are contaminated with the bacterium Listeria monocytogenes. Pregnant women are at an increased risk of contracting listeriosis and experiencing severe illness as a result. To reduce the risk of listeriosis, pregnant women should thoroughly wash and properly store vegetables, and should avoid consuming vegetables that are past their expiration date or have an off smell or taste.

Overall, cauliflower can be a nutritious and enjoyable part of a healthy diet during pregnancy when consumed in moderation and with appropriate precautions. As with any food, it is important for pregnant women to speak with their healthcare provider about their dietary needs and any potential risks or concerns.

Cauliflower rice

Cauliflower rice is a type of dish that is made by grating or processing cauliflower into small, rice-like pieces. It is often used as a lower-carbohydrate alternative to rice or as a way to add more vegetables to the diet.

Cauliflower rice is a good source of dietary fiber, vitamins, and minerals, including vitamin C, vitamin K, and potassium. These nutrients are important for fetal development and the health of the mother during pregnancy.

Cauliflower rice is also low in calories and fat, making it a healthy and nutritious addition to the diet of a pregnant woman. It is a good idea to choose cauliflower rice that is made with minimal amounts of added sugars and unhealthy fats, and to limit the intake of added sugars and unhealthy fats during pregnancy.

In addition, it is important to follow proper food safety guidelines when consuming cauliflower rice or any other food during pregnancy. This includes washing the ingredients thoroughly to remove any dirt or contaminants, and discarding any cauliflower rice that is spoiled or shows signs of spoilage.

Overall, cauliflower rice can be a healthy and nutritious addition to the diet of a pregnant woman, as long as it is consumed in moderation as part of a balanced diet. It is a good idea to consult with a healthcare provider or a registered dietitian for personalized nutrition advice.

Cheddar cheese

Cheddar cheese is a type of hard, yellow or white cheese with a sharp, tangy flavor. It is made from cow's milk and is a good source of protein, calcium, and other nutrients. Cheddar cheese is generally considered safe to consume during pregnancy when prepared and consumed properly.

Eating a variety of dairy products, including cheddar cheese, during pregnancy can provide important nutrients and contribute to a healthy diet. However, it is important for pregnant women to be mindful of the risk of contracting foodborne illness, as they are at an increased risk of severe illness as a result of certain types of infections.

To reduce the risk of foodborne illness, pregnant women should thoroughly wash and properly store fresh produce, and should avoid consuming produce that is past its expiration date or has an off smell or taste. Pregnant women should also be careful to fully cook cheddar cheese and other dairy products to kill any harmful bacteria that may be present.

In addition, pregnant women should be aware of the risk of contracting listeriosis, a bacterial infection that can be caused by consuming contaminated food. Cheddar cheese and other dairy products can be a source of listeriosis if they are contaminated with the bacterium Listeria monocytogenes. Pregnant women are at an increased risk of contracting listeriosis and experiencing severe illness as a result. To reduce the risk of listeriosis, pregnant women should thoroughly wash and properly store dairy products, and should avoid consuming dairy products that are past their expiration date or have an off smell or taste.

Overall, cheddar cheese can be a nutritious and enjoyable part of a healthy diet during pregnancy when consumed in moderation and with appropriate precautions. As with any food, it is important for pregnant women to speak with their healthcare provider about their dietary needs and any potential risks or concerns.

Cereal bars

Cereal bars are a type of snack that is made with cereal grains, sugar, and other ingredients. While they can be a convenient snack option, it is important to choose cereal bars that are nutritious and safe to eat during pregnancy.

Many store-bought and homemade cereal bars are high in added sugars, salt, and unhealthy fats, and provide little nutritional value. These types of cereal bars can contribute to weight gain and increase the risk of gestational diabetes and other pregnancy complications.

It is a good idea to choose cereal bars that are made with healthier ingredients, such as whole grain cereals, natural sweeteners, and minimal amounts of salt and unhealthy fats, and to limit the intake of added sugars and unhealthy fats. You can also make your own cereal bars at home using healthier ingredients, such as whole grain cereals, natural sweeteners, and unsweetened fruit or nut butter, to control the nutritional content of the bars.

In addition, it is important to follow proper food safety guidelines when consuming cereal bars or any other food during pregnancy. This includes checking the expiration date and discarding any cereal bars that are spoiled or show signs of spoilage.

Overall, it is a good idea to choose cereal bars that are nutritious and safe to eat during pregnancy, and to consume them in moderation as part of a balanced diet. It is a good idea to consult with a healthcare provider or a registered dietitian for personalized nutrition advice.

Chiropractic care

Chiropractic care is a form of alternative medicine that focuses on the diagnosis and treatment of neuromuscular disorders. Chiropractic care is based on the belief that the body has the ability to heal itself and that proper alignment of the musculoskeletal structure, particularly the spine, can contribute to overall health and well-being.

There is limited research on the safety and effectiveness of chiropractic care during pregnancy. Some studies have suggested that chiropractic care may be safe and beneficial for pregnant women, while others have not found significant benefits.

The American Pregnancy Association (APA) recommends that pregnant women consult with their healthcare provider before seeking chiropractic care. The APA also recommends that pregnant women choose a chiropractor who is experienced in working with pregnant women and who uses techniques that are specifically designed for pregnancy.

It is important for pregnant women to be aware that chiropractic care may not be appropriate for everyone and that it should not be used as a substitute for medical care. Pregnant women who are considering chiropractic care should speak with their healthcare provider about their individual needs and any potential risks or concerns.

Chocolate

Chocolate is a food product made from the seeds of the cocoa tree. It is a source of cocoa butter, cocoa solids, sugar, and milk, and is available in a variety of forms, including solid chocolate bars, chocolate chips, and chocolate-flavored beverages. Chocolate is a popular treat that is enjoyed by many people around the world.

During pregnancy, it is generally considered safe to consume chocolate in moderation. Chocolate is a source of antioxidants and other nutrients, and it may have some potential health benefits when consumed in moderation. However, it is important for pregnant women to be aware of the potential risks of consuming chocolate, as well as the potential benefits.

One potential risk of consuming chocolate during pregnancy is the risk of consuming too much caffeine. Chocolate contains caffeine, which is a stimulant that can affect the central nervous system. The recommended daily intake of caffeine for pregnant women is 200 milligrams per day or less. Consuming more than this amount of caffeine during pregnancy may increase the risk of certain complications, such as preterm birth and low birth weight. It is important for pregnant women to be aware of the caffeine content of the foods and beverages they consume, and to speak with their healthcare provider about their caffeine intake and any potential risks or concerns.

In addition, chocolate is high in calories and can contribute to weight gain if consumed in excess. Pregnant women who are concerned about their weight should be mindful of their chocolate intake and choose chocolate products in moderation.

Overall, chocolate can be a nutritious and enjoyable part of a healthy diet during pregnancy when consumed in moderation and with appropriate precautions. As with any food, it is important for pregnant women to speak with their healthcare provider about their dietary needs and any potential risks or concerns.

Chocolate chips

Chocolate chips are small pieces of chocolate that are often used in baking and cooking. While they can be a tasty and indulgent ingredient, it is important to choose chocolate chips that are nutritious and safe to eat during pregnancy.

Many store-bought and homemade chocolate chips are high in added sugars, unhealthy fats, and calories, and provide little nutritional value. These types of chocolate chips can contribute to weight gain and increase the risk of gestational diabetes and other pregnancy complications.

It is a good idea to choose chocolate chips that are made with healthier ingredients, such as cocoa, natural sweeteners, and minimal amounts of unhealthy fats, and to limit the intake of added sugars and unhealthy fats. You can also make your own chocolate chips at home using healthier ingredients, such as cocoa, natural sweeteners, and unsweetened fruit or nut butter, to control the nutritional content of the chocolate chips.

In addition, it is important to follow proper food safety guidelines when consuming chocolate chips or any other food during pregnancy. This includes checking the expiration date and discarding any chocolate chips that are spoiled or show signs of spoilage.

Overall, it is a good idea to choose chocolate chips that are nutritious and safe to eat during pregnancy, and to consume them in moderation as part of a balanced diet. It is a good idea to consult with a healthcare provider or a registered dietitian for personalized nutrition advice.

Chocolate milk

Chocolate milk is a type of milk that is flavored with cocoa or chocolate syrup. While it can be a tasty and convenient drink option, it is important to choose chocolate milk that is nutritious and safe to eat during pregnancy.

Many store-bought and homemade chocolate milks are high in added sugars, unhealthy fats, and calories, and provide little nutritional value. These types of chocolate milks can contribute to weight gain and increase the risk of gestational diabetes and other pregnancy complications.

It is a good idea to choose chocolate milk that is made with healthier ingredients, such as low-fat or reduced-fat milk, cocoa, natural sweeteners, and minimal amounts of unhealthy fats, and to limit the intake of added sugars and unhealthy fats. You can also make your own chocolate milk at home using healthier ingredients, such as low-fat or reduced-fat milk, cocoa, natural sweeteners, and unsweetened fruit or nut butter, to control the nutritional content of the chocolate milk.

In addition, it is important to follow proper food safety guidelines when consuming chocolate milk or any other food during pregnancy. This includes checking the expiration date and discarding any chocolate milk that is spoiled or shows signs of spoilage.

Overall, it is a good idea to choose chocolate milk that is nutritious and safe to eat during pregnancy, and to consume it in moderation as part of a balanced diet. It is a good idea to consult with a healthcare provider or a registered dietitian for personalized nutrition advice.

Chutney

Chutney is a type of condiment that is made with fruit, vinegar, sugar, and spices. While it can be a tasty and convenient condiment option, it is important to choose chutney that is nutritious and safe to eat during pregnancy.

Many store-bought and homemade chutneys are high in salt, added sugars, and unhealthy fats, and provide little nutritional value. These types of chutneys can contribute to weight gain and increase the risk of gestational diabetes and other pregnancy complications.

It is a good idea to choose chutney that is made with healthier ingredients, such as fruit, vinegar, natural sweeteners, and minimal amounts of salt and unhealthy fats, and to limit the intake of added sugars and unhealthy fats. You can also make your own chutney at home using healthier ingredients, such as fruit, vinegar, natural sweeteners, and unsweetened fruit or nut butter, to control the nutritional content of the chutney.

In addition, it is important to follow proper food safety guidelines when consuming chutney or any other food during pregnancy. This includes washing the ingredients thoroughly to remove any dirt or contaminants, and discarding any chutney that is spoiled or shows signs of spoilage.

Overall, it is a good idea to choose chutney that is nutritious and safe to eat during pregnancy, and to consume it in moderation as part of a balanced diet. It is a good idea to consult with a healthcare provider or a registered dietitian for personalized nutrition advice.

Clam chowder

Clam chowder is a type of soup that is made with clams, potatoes, and other vegetables in a creamy broth. While it can be a tasty and satisfying meal option, it is important to choose clam chowder that is nutritious and safe to eat during pregnancy.

Many store-bought and homemade clam chowders are high in salt, added sugars, and unhealthy fats, and provide little nutritional value. These types of clam chowders can contribute to weight gain and increase the risk of gestational diabetes and other pregnancy complications.

It is a good idea to choose clam chowder that is made with healthier ingredients, such as clams, potatoes, vegetables, and minimal amounts of salt and unhealthy fats, and to limit the intake of added sugars and unhealthy fats. You can also make your own clam chowder at home using healthier ingredients, such as clams, potatoes, vegetables, and unsweetened fruit or nut butter, to control the nutritional content of the clam chowder.

In addition, it is important to follow proper food safety guidelines when consuming clam chowder or any other food during pregnancy. This includes washing the ingredients thoroughly to remove any dirt or contaminants, and discarding any clam chowder that is spoiled or shows signs of spoilage.

Overall, it is a good idea to choose clam chowder that is nutritious and safe to eat during pregnancy, and to consume it in moderation as part of a balanced diet. It is a good idea to consult with a healthcare provider or a registered dietitian for personalized nutrition advice.

Coconut milk

Coconut milk is a type of milk that is made from the flesh of coconuts. While it can be a tasty and convenient drink option, it is important to choose coconut milk that is nutritious and safe to eat during pregnancy.

Many store-bought and homemade coconut milks are high in added sugars, unhealthy fats, and calories, and provide little nutritional value. These types of coconut milks can contribute to weight gain and increase the risk of gestational diabetes and other pregnancy complications.

It is a good idea to choose coconut milk that is made with healthier ingredients, such as coconut, natural sweeteners, and minimal amounts of unhealthy fats, and to limit the intake of added sugars and unhealthy fats. You can also make your own coconut milk at home using healthier ingredients, such as coconut, natural sweeteners, and unsweetened fruit or nut butter, to control the nutritional content of the coconut milk.

In addition, it is important to follow proper food safety guidelines when consuming coconut milk or any other food during pregnancy. This includes checking the expiration date and discarding any coconut milk that is spoiled or shows signs of spoilage.

Overall, it is a good idea to choose coconut milk that is nutritious and safe to eat during pregnancy, and to consume it in moderation as part of a balanced diet. It is a good idea to consult with a

healthcare provider or a registered dietitian for personalized nutrition advice.

Coffee

Caffeine is a stimulant that is found in a variety of beverages and foods, including coffee, tea, soda, chocolate, and some medications. While caffeine is generally considered safe to consume in moderation, pregnant women may need to be cautious about their caffeine intake.

During pregnancy, caffeine can cross the placenta and reach the baby. High levels of caffeine in the mother's bloodstream may affect the baby's heart rate and sleep patterns. Some studies have also suggested that consuming high levels of caffeine during pregnancy may increase the risk of miscarriage and low birth weight.

The American College of Obstetricians and Gynecologists (ACOG) recommends that pregnant women limit their caffeine intake to 200 milligrams (mg) or less per day. This is equivalent to about one or two 8-ounce cups of coffee. It is important to note that the caffeine content of beverages and foods can vary widely, so it is important for pregnant women to be aware of the sources of caffeine in their diet.

It is also worth noting that some studies have suggested that consuming moderate amounts of caffeine during pregnancy may not be harmful. However, the potential risks of consuming high levels of caffeine during pregnancy are not fully understood, and it is generally recommended that pregnant women err on the side of caution and limit their caffeine intake.

Pregnant women who are concerned about their caffeine intake should discuss their concerns with their healthcare provider. It is also a good idea for pregnant women to pay attention to the other sources of caffeine in their diet, such as chocolate, tea, and certain medications.

In summary, while caffeine is generally considered safe to consume in moderation, pregnant women should be cautious about their caffeine intake and aim to limit their intake to 200 mg or less per day. Pregnant women who are concerned about their caffeine intake should discuss their concerns with their healthcare provider.

Coffee creamer

Coffee creamer is a type of dairy or non-dairy product that is used to add flavor and creaminess to coffee. While it can be a tasty and convenient way to enhance the flavor of coffee, it is important to choose coffee creamer that is nutritious and safe to eat during pregnancy.

Many store-bought and homemade coffee creamers are high in added sugars, unhealthy fats, and calories, and provide little nutritional value. These types of coffee creamers can contribute to weight gain and increase the risk of gestational diabetes and other pregnancy complications.

It is a good idea to choose coffee creamer that is made with healthier ingredients, such as low-fat or reduced-fat milk, natural sweeteners, and minimal amounts of unhealthy fats, and to limit the intake of added sugars and unhealthy fats. You can also make your own coffee creamer at home using healthier ingredients, such as low-fat or reduced-fat milk, natural sweeteners, and unsweetened fruit or nut butter, to control the nutritional content of the coffee creamer.

In addition, it is important to follow proper food safety guidelines when consuming coffee creamer or any other food during pregnancy. This includes checking the expiration date and discarding any coffee creamer that is spoiled or shows signs of spoilage.

Overall, it is a good idea to choose coffee creamer that is nutritious and safe to eat during pregnancy, and to consume it in moderation as part of a balanced diet. It is a good idea to consult with a

healthcare provider or a registered dietitian for personalized nutrition advice.

Collard greens

Collard greens are a type of leafy green vegetable that is rich in nutrients and has a slightly bitter and slightly sweet taste. They are a good source of fiber, vitamins, minerals, and antioxidants, and can be a nutritious and safe food to eat during pregnancy.

Collard greens are a good source of vitamin C, vitamin K, vitamin A, calcium, and folate, which are important nutrients for pregnancy. Vitamin C helps to support the immune system and promote healthy skin, while vitamin K is important for blood clotting and bone health. Vitamin A supports eye health and the development of the fetal organs, while calcium is important for the development of strong bones and teeth. Folate is important for the proper development of the neural tube, which becomes the brain and spinal cord.

In addition, collard greens are a good source of antioxidants, which can help to reduce the risk of chronic diseases and support overall health.

It is a good idea to consume collard greens as part of a balanced diet during pregnancy, along with other nutrient-rich foods. Collard greens can be cooked in a variety of ways, such as steamed, sautéed, braised, or boiled, and can be added to soups, stews, casseroles, or used as a wrap for sandwiches.

It is important to follow proper food safety guidelines when consuming collard greens or any other food during pregnancy. This includes washing the collard greens thoroughly to remove any dirt or contaminants, and discarding any collard greens that are spoiled or show signs of spoilage.

Overall, collard greens can be a nutritious and safe food to eat during pregnancy, and it is a good idea to consult with a healthcare provider or a registered dietitian for personalized nutrition advice.

Constipation relief products

Constipation is a common digestive problem that is characterized by infrequent or difficult bowel movements. It can be caused by a variety of factors, including a low-fiber diet, insufficient fluid intake, and certain medications. Constipation can be uncomfortable and may cause abdominal pain, bloating, and difficulty passing stools.

During pregnancy, constipation is a common issue, as the growing uterus can put pressure on the intestines and cause bowel movements to slow down. Constipation relief products are medications or other products that are designed to help alleviate constipation.

There are a variety of constipation relief products available, including over-the-counter (OTC) medications, such as fiber supplements, stool softeners, and laxatives, and prescription medications. It is important for pregnant women to speak with their healthcare provider before using any constipation relief products, as some products may not be safe for use during pregnancy.

The safety and effectiveness of constipation relief products during pregnancy can vary depending on the specific product and the individual circumstances of the pregnant woman. Some OTC constipation relief products, such as fiber supplements and stool softeners, are generally considered safe for use during pregnancy when used as directed. However, other products, such as stimulant laxatives, may not be recommended for use during pregnancy.

It is important for pregnant women to speak with their healthcare provider about the best approach to relieving constipation and to follow their recommendations. Pregnant women who are experiencing constipation may also be able to relieve symptoms by increasing their intake of fluids and fiber, exercising regularly, and avoiding straining during bowel movements.

Coping strategies for stress and anxiety

Pregnancy can be a time of emotional and physical changes, and it is normal for pregnant women to experience some stress and anxiety. Coping strategies are techniques or approaches that can help individuals manage stress and anxiety.

There are a variety of coping strategies that pregnant women can use to manage stress and anxiety, including:

1. Exercise: Regular physical activity can help reduce stress and improve overall well-being. Pregnant women should consult with their healthcare provider before starting or continuing an exercise program.

2. Relaxation techniques: Techniques such as deep breathing, progressive muscle relaxation, and meditation can help reduce stress and promote relaxation.

3. Social support: Surrounding oneself with supportive friends and family members can help reduce stress and improve overall well-being.

4. Time management: Planning and organizing tasks and responsibilities can help reduce stress and improve productivity.

5. Self-care: Taking care of one's physical and emotional well-being, including getting enough sleep, eating a healthy diet, and engaging in activities that bring joy and relaxation, can help reduce stress and improve overall well-being.

6. Professional help: Seeking the help of a mental health professional, such as a therapist or counselor, can be an effective way to manage stress and anxiety.

It is important for pregnant women to find coping strategies that work for them and to speak with their healthcare provider if they are struggling to manage stress and anxiety.

Corn

Corn is a type of cereal grain that is widely cultivated for its edible seeds. It is a staple food in many parts of the world and is available in a variety of forms, including fresh, frozen, canned, and dried. Corn is a good source of nutrients, including vitamins, minerals, and fiber. Corn is generally considered safe to consume during pregnancy when prepared and consumed properly.

Eating a variety of grains, including corn, during pregnancy can provide important nutrients and contribute to a healthy diet. However, it is important for pregnant women to be mindful of the risk of contracting foodborne illness, as they are at an increased risk of severe illness as a result of certain types of infections.

To reduce the risk of foodborne illness, pregnant women should thoroughly wash and properly store fresh produce, and should avoid consuming produce that is past its expiration date or has an off smell or taste. Pregnant women should also be careful to fully cook corn and other grains to kill any harmful bacteria that may be present.

In addition, pregnant women should be aware of the risk of contracting listeriosis, a bacterial infection that can be caused by consuming contaminated food. Corn and other grains can be a source of listeriosis if they are contaminated with the bacterium Listeria monocytogenes. Pregnant women are at an increased risk of contracting listeriosis and experiencing severe illness as a result. To reduce the risk of listeriosis, pregnant women should thoroughly wash and properly store grains, and should avoid consuming grains that are past their expiration date or have an off smell or taste.

Overall, corn can be a nutritious and enjoyable part of a healthy diet during pregnancy when consumed in moderation and with appropriate precautions. As with any food, it is important for pregnant women to speak with their healthcare provider about their dietary needs and any potential risks or concerns.

Cornbread

Cornbread is a type of bread that is made with cornmeal, flour, and other ingredients. While it can be a tasty and convenient bread option, it is important to choose cornbread that is nutritious and safe to eat during pregnancy.

Many store-bought and homemade cornbreads are high in added sugars, unhealthy fats, and calories, and provide little nutritional value. These types of cornbreads can contribute to weight gain and increase the risk of gestational diabetes and other pregnancy complications.

It is a good idea to choose cornbread that is made with healthier ingredients, such as cornmeal, whole grain flour, natural sweeteners, and minimal amounts of unhealthy fats, and to limit the intake of added sugars and unhealthy fats. You can also make your own cornbread at home using healthier ingredients, such as cornmeal, whole grain flour, natural sweeteners, and unsweetened fruit or nut butter, to control the nutritional content of the cornbread.

In addition, it is important to follow proper food safety guidelines when consuming cornbread or any other food during pregnancy. This includes checking the expiration date and discarding any cornbread that is spoiled or shows signs of spoilage.

Overall, it is a good idea to choose cornbread that is nutritious and safe to eat during pregnancy, and to consume it in moderation as part of a balanced diet. It is a good idea to consult with a healthcare provider or a registered dietitian for personalized nutrition advice.

Corned beef

Corned beef is a type of beef that is cured with salt and spices and is often served as a sandwich meat or in dishes such as corned beef hash. While it can be a tasty and convenient protein option, it is important to choose corned beef that is nutritious and safe to eat during pregnancy.

Many store-bought and homemade corned beefs are high in salt, added sugars, and unhealthy fats, and provide little nutritional value. These types of corned beefs can contribute to weight gain and increase the risk of gestational diabetes and other pregnancy complications.

It is a good idea to choose corned beef that is made with healthier ingredients, such as beef, natural spices, and minimal amounts of salt and unhealthy fats, and to limit the intake of added sugars and unhealthy fats. You can also make your own corned beef at home using healthier ingredients, such as beef, natural spices, and unsweetened fruit or nut butter, to control the nutritional content of the corned beef.

In addition, it is important to follow proper food safety guidelines when consuming corned beef or any other food during pregnancy. This includes washing the ingredients thoroughly to remove any dirt or contaminants, and discarding any corned beef that is spoiled or shows signs of spoilage.

Overall, it is a good idea to choose corned beef that is nutritious and safe to eat during pregnancy, and to consume it in moderation as part of a balanced diet. It is a good idea to consult with a healthcare provider or a registered dietitian for personalized nutrition advice.

Cottage cheese

Cottage cheese is a type of cheese made from the curds of cow's milk. It has a soft, creamy texture and a mild, slightly tangy flavor. Cottage cheese is a good source of protein, calcium, and other nutrients. Cottage cheese is generally considered safe to consume during pregnancy when prepared and consumed properly.

Eating a variety of dairy products, including cottage cheese, during pregnancy can provide important nutrients and contribute to a healthy diet. However, it is important for pregnant women to be mindful of the risk of contracting foodborne illness, as they are at an increased risk of severe illness as a result of certain types of infections.

To reduce the risk of foodborne illness, pregnant women should thoroughly wash and properly store fresh produce, and should avoid consuming produce that is past its expiration date or has an off smell or taste. Pregnant women should also be careful to fully cook cottage cheese and other dairy products to kill any harmful bacteria that may be present.

In addition, pregnant women should be aware of the risk of contracting listeriosis, a bacterial infection that can be caused by consuming contaminated food. Cottage cheese and other dairy products can be a source of listeriosis if they are contaminated with the bacterium Listeria monocytogenes. Pregnant women are at an increased risk of contracting listeriosis and experiencing severe illness as a result. To reduce the risk of listeriosis, pregnant women should thoroughly wash and properly store dairy products, and should avoid consuming dairy products that are past their expiration date or have an off smell or taste.

Overall, cottage cheese can be a nutritious and enjoyable part of a healthy diet during pregnancy when consumed in moderation and with appropriate precautions. As with any food, it is important for pregnant women to speak with their healthcare provider about their dietary needs and any potential risks or concerns.

Crab cakes

Crab cakes are a type of food that is made with crab meat, bread crumbs, and other ingredients and is often served as an appetizer or main dish. While they can be a tasty and convenient food option, it is important to choose crab cakes that are nutritious and safe to eat during pregnancy.

Many store-bought and homemade crab cakes are high in added sugars, unhealthy fats, and calories, and provide little nutritional value. These types of crab cakes can contribute to weight gain and increase the risk of gestational diabetes and other pregnancy complications.

It is a good idea to choose crab cakes that are made with healthier ingredients, such as crab meat, whole grain bread crumbs, natural sweeteners, and minimal amounts of unhealthy fats, and to limit the intake of added sugars and unhealthy fats. You can also make your own crab cakes at home using healthier ingredients, such as crab meat, whole grain bread crumbs, natural sweeteners, and unsweetened fruit or nut butter, to control the nutritional content of the crab cakes.

In addition, it is important to follow proper food safety guidelines when consuming crab cakes or any other food during pregnancy. This includes washing the ingredients thoroughly to remove any dirt or contaminants, and discarding any crab cakes that are spoiled or show signs of spoilage.

Overall, it is a good idea to choose crab cakes that are nutritious and safe to eat during pregnancy, and to consume them in moderation as part of a balanced diet. It is a good idea to consult with a healthcare provider or a registered dietitian for personalized nutrition advice.

Crackers

Crackers are small, thin, crisp baked goods that are made from flour, water, and other ingredients. They are often flavored with spices, herbs, seeds, or cheese, and are available in a variety of shapes and sizes. Crackers are a popular snack that is enjoyed by many people around the world.

During pregnancy, it is generally considered safe to consume crackers in moderation. Crackers are a good source of carbohydrates, which provide energy and are an important part of a healthy diet. However, it is important for pregnant women to be aware of the potential risks of consuming crackers, as well as the potential benefits.

One potential risk of consuming crackers during pregnancy is the risk of consuming too much sodium. Some crackers are high in sodium, which can contribute to high blood pressure, a common complication of pregnancy. It is important for pregnant women to be mindful of the sodium content of the foods and beverages they consume and to choose crackers that are lower in sodium.

In addition, crackers are often high in calories and may contribute to weight gain if consumed in excess. Pregnant women who are concerned about their weight should be mindful of their cracker intake and choose crackers in moderation.

Overall, crackers can be a nutritious and enjoyable part of a healthy diet during pregnancy when consumed in moderation and with appropriate precautions. As with any food, it is important for pregnant women to speak with their healthcare provider about their dietary needs and any potential risks or concerns.

Cranberry sauce

Cranberry sauce is a type of condiment that is made with cranberries, sugar, and other ingredients and is often served with Thanksgiving or Christmas dinners. While it can be a tasty and convenient condiment option, it is important to choose cranberry sauce that is nutritious and safe to eat during pregnancy.

Many store-bought and homemade cranberry sauces are high in added sugars and calories, and provide little nutritional value. These types of cranberry sauces can contribute to weight gain and increase the risk of gestational diabetes and other pregnancy complications.

It is a good idea to choose cranberry sauce that is made with healthier ingredients, such as cranberries, natural sweeteners, and minimal amounts of unhealthy fats, and to limit the intake of added sugars. You can also make your own cranberry sauce at home using healthier ingredients, such as cranberries, natural sweeteners, and unsweetened fruit or nut butter, to control the nutritional content of the cranberry sauce.

In addition, it is important to follow proper food safety guidelines when consuming cranberry sauce or any other food during pregnancy. This includes checking the expiration date and discarding any cranberry sauce that is spoiled or shows signs of spoilage.

Overall, it is a good idea to choose cranberry sauce that is nutritious and safe to eat during pregnancy, and to consume it in moderation as part of a balanced diet. It is a good idea to consult with a healthcare provider or a registered dietitian for personalized nutrition advice.

Cream cheese

Cream cheese is a type of cheese that is made with milk and cream and has a soft and creamy texture. While it can be a tasty and convenient cheese option, it is important to choose cream cheese that is nutritious and safe to eat during pregnancy.

Many store-bought and homemade cream cheeses are high in unhealthy fats, added sugars, and calories, and provide little nutritional value. These types of cream cheeses can contribute to weight gain and increase the risk of gestational diabetes and other pregnancy complications.

It is a good idea to choose cream cheese that is made with healthier ingredients, such as low-fat or reduced-fat milk and cream, natural sweeteners, and minimal amounts of unhealthy fats, and to limit the intake of added sugars and unhealthy fats. You can also make your own cream cheese at home using healthier ingredients, such as low-fat or reduced-fat milk and cream, natural sweeteners, and unsweetened fruit or nut butter, to control the nutritional content of the cream cheese.

In addition, it is important to follow proper food safety guidelines when consuming cream cheese or any other food during pregnancy. This includes checking the expiration date and discarding any cream cheese that is spoiled or shows signs of spoilage.

Overall, it is a good idea to choose cream cheese that is nutritious and safe to eat during pregnancy, and to consume it in moderation as part of a balanced diet. It is a good idea to consult with a healthcare provider or a registered dietitian for personalized nutrition advice.

Cream of mushroom soup

Cream of mushroom soup is a type of soup that is made with mushrooms, milk or cream, and other ingredients and has a creamy and smooth texture. While it can be a tasty and convenient soup option, it is important to choose cream of mushroom soup that is nutritious and safe to eat during pregnancy.

Many store-bought and homemade cream of mushroom soups are high in unhealthy fats, added sugars, and sodium, and provide little nutritional value. These types of cream of mushroom soups can contribute to weight gain and increase the risk of gestational diabetes and other pregnancy complications.

It is a good idea to choose cream of mushroom soup that is made with healthier ingredients, such as mushrooms, low-fat or reduced-fat milk or cream, natural sweeteners, and minimal amounts of unhealthy fats and sodium, and to limit the intake of added sugars and unhealthy fats. You can also make your own cream of mushroom soup at home using healthier ingredients, such as mushrooms, low-fat or reduced-fat milk or cream, natural sweeteners, and unsweetened fruit or nut butter, to control the nutritional content of the cream of mushroom soup.

In addition, it is important to follow proper food safety guidelines when consuming cream of mushroom soup or any other food during pregnancy. This includes checking the expiration date and discarding any cream of mushroom soup that is spoiled or shows signs of spoilage.

Overall, it is a good idea to choose cream of mushroom soup that is nutritious and safe to eat during pregnancy, and to consume it in moderation as part of a balanced diet. It is a good idea to consult with a healthcare provider or a registered dietitian for personalized nutrition advice.

Creamed spinach

Creamed spinach is a type of dish that is made with spinach, milk or cream, and other ingredients and has a creamy and smooth texture. While it can be a tasty and convenient dish option, it is important to choose creamed spinach that is nutritious and safe to eat during pregnancy.

Many store-bought and homemade creamed spinaches are high in unhealthy fats, added sugars, and sodium, and provide little nutritional value. These types of creamed spinaches can contribute to weight gain and increase the risk of gestational diabetes and other pregnancy complications.

It is a good idea to choose creamed spinach that is made with healthier ingredients, such as spinach, low-fat or reduced-fat milk or cream, natural sweeteners, and minimal amounts of unhealthy fats and sodium, and to limit the intake of added sugars and unhealthy fats. You can also make your own creamed spinach at home using healthier ingredients, such as spinach, low-fat or reduced-fat milk or cream, natural sweeteners, and unsweetened fruit or nut butter, to control the nutritional content of the creamed spinach.

In addition, it is important to follow proper food safety guidelines when consuming creamed spinach or any other food during pregnancy. This includes washing the ingredients thoroughly to remove any dirt or contaminants, and discarding any creamed spinach that is spoiled or shows signs of spoilage.

Overall, it is a good idea to choose creamed spinach that is nutritious and safe to eat during pregnancy, and to consume it in moderation as part of a balanced diet. It is a good idea to consult with a

healthcare provider or a registered dietitian for personalized nutrition advice.

Creole seasoning

Creole seasoning is a type of spice blend that is commonly used in Creole cuisine, which is a style of cooking that originated in New Orleans, Louisiana. Creole seasoning is typically made with a combination of herbs and spices, such as paprika, garlic, onion, and chili pepper, and is often used to add flavor to a variety of dishes, including meats, seafood, and vegetables.

During pregnancy, it is generally considered safe to consume Creole seasoning as part of a healthy diet. Creole seasoning is a good source of nutrients, including vitamins and minerals, and may have potential health benefits. However, it is important for pregnant women to be aware of the potential risks of consuming Creole seasoning, as well as the potential benefits.

Some pregnant women may be allergic to certain herbs or spices that are used in Creole seasoning or may have sensitivities to them. In addition, consuming large amounts of Creole seasoning may cause heartburn or other digestive problems in some individuals.

It is generally recommended for pregnant women to consume Creole seasoning in moderation and to speak with their healthcare provider if they are concerned about the potential risks of consuming Creole seasoning. Pregnant women should also be aware of any food allergies or sensitivities they may have and should speak with their healthcare provider if they are concerned about the potential risks of consuming Creole seasoning.

Overall, Creole seasoning can be a flavorful part of a healthy diet during pregnancy when consumed in moderation and with appropriate precautions. Pregnant women should speak with their healthcare provider about their dietary needs and any potential risks or concerns.

Crispy chicken sandwich

A crispy chicken sandwich is a type of sandwich that typically consists of breaded and fried chicken that is served on a bun or other type of bread, along with various toppings, such as lettuce, tomato, cheese, and mayonnaise.

During pregnancy, it is generally considered safe to consume a crispy chicken sandwich as part of a healthy diet. Chicken is a good source of protein, which is important for the growth and development of the fetus and for the maintenance of the pregnant woman's tissues. Bread is a good source of carbohydrates, which provide energy to the body, and vegetables, such as lettuce and tomato, are a good source of nutrients, including vitamins and minerals.

However, it is important for pregnant women to be aware of the potential risks of consuming a crispy chicken sandwich, as well as the potential benefits. Some pregnant women may be allergic to chicken or may have sensitivities to it. In addition, consuming large amounts of fried foods may increase the risk of heart disease and other health problems.

It is generally recommended for pregnant women to consume a crispy chicken sandwich in moderation and to speak with their healthcare provider if they are concerned about the potential risks of consuming a crispy chicken sandwich. Pregnant women should also be aware of any food allergies or sensitivities they may have and should speak with their healthcare provider if they are concerned about the potential risks of consuming a crispy chicken sandwich.

Overall, a crispy chicken sandwich can be a tasty and convenient part of a healthy diet during pregnancy when consumed in moderation and with appropriate precautions. Pregnant women should speak with their healthcare provider about their dietary needs and any potential risks or concerns.

Croissants

Croissants are a type of pastry that is made with layers of butter and dough that are rolled and folded to create a flaky, crescent-shaped pastry. Croissants are often served as a breakfast or snack food and may be filled with various ingredients, such as jam, chocolate, or cheese.

During pregnancy, it is generally considered safe to consume croissants as part of a healthy diet. Croissants are a good source of carbohydrates, which provide energy to the body, and may have potential health benefits. However, it is important for pregnant women to be aware of the potential risks of consuming croissants, as well as the potential benefits.

Some pregnant women may be allergic to croissants or may have sensitivities to them. In addition, consuming large amounts of croissants may increase the risk of weight gain and other health problems. Croissants are also typically high in calories, fat, and sugar, which may not be suitable for pregnant women who are trying to manage their weight or blood sugar levels.

It is generally recommended for pregnant women to consume croissants in moderation and to speak with their healthcare provider if they are concerned about the potential risks of consuming croissants. Pregnant women should also be aware of any food allergies or sensitivities they may have and should speak with their healthcare provider if they are concerned about the potential risks of consuming croissants.

Overall, croissants can be a tasty and convenient part of a healthy diet during pregnancy when consumed in moderation and with appropriate precautions. Pregnant women should speak with their healthcare provider about their dietary needs and any potential risks or concerns.

Cupcakes

Cupcakes are small, individual-sized cakes that are baked in a muffin tin and are often topped with frosting or other types of decorations. Cupcakes are a popular dessert option and may be flavored with various ingredients, such as chocolate, vanilla, or fruit.

During pregnancy, it is generally considered safe to consume cupcakes as part of a healthy diet. Cupcakes are a good source of carbohydrates, which provide energy to the body, and may have potential health benefits. However, it is important for pregnant women to be aware of the potential risks of consuming cupcakes, as well as the potential benefits.

Some pregnant women may be allergic to cupcakes or may have sensitivities to them. In addition, consuming large amounts of cupcakes may increase the risk of weight gain and other health problems. Cupcakes are also typically high in calories, fat, and sugar, which may not be suitable for pregnant women who are trying to manage their weight or blood sugar levels.

It is generally recommended for pregnant women to consume cupcakes in moderation and to speak with their healthcare provider if they are concerned about the potential risks of consuming cupcakes. Pregnant women should also be aware of any food allergies or sensitivities they may have and should speak with their healthcare provider if they are concerned about the potential risks of consuming cupcakes.

Overall, cupcakes can be a tasty and convenient part of a healthy diet during pregnancy when consumed in moderation and with appropriate precautions. Pregnant women should speak with their healthcare provider about their dietary needs and any potential risks or concerns.

Curry

Curry is a type of dish that is typically made with a blend of spices, herbs, and other ingredients and is often served with rice or other grains. Curry dishes may be made with a variety of meats, vegetables, and legumes, and may be flavored with various types of sauces or pastes.

During pregnancy, it is generally considered safe to consume curry as part of a healthy diet. Curry is a good source of nutrients, including vitamins and minerals, and may have potential health benefits. However, it is important for pregnant women to be aware of the potential risks of consuming curry, as well as the potential benefits.

Some pregnant women may be allergic to curry or may have sensitivities to it. In addition, consuming large amounts of curry may cause heartburn or other digestive problems in some individuals. Curry may also contain high levels of sodium or other ingredients that may not be suitable for pregnant women who are trying to manage their blood pressure or other health conditions.

It is generally recommended for pregnant women to consume curry in moderation and to speak with their healthcare provider if they are concerned about the potential risks of consuming curry. Pregnant women should also be aware of any food allergies or sensitivities they may have and should speak with their healthcare provider if they are concerned about the potential risks of consuming curry.

Overall, curry can be a flavorful and nutritious part of a healthy diet during pregnancy when consumed in moderation and with appropriate precautions. Pregnant women should speak with their healthcare provider about their dietary needs and any potential risks or concerns.

Dates

Dates are a type of dried fruit that is native to the Middle East and North Africa. They are sweet, chewy, and nutritionally dense, and are available in a variety of shapes, sizes, and colors. Dates are a good source of a variety of nutrients, including fiber, potassium, and antioxidants.

During pregnancy, it is generally considered safe to consume dates in moderation. Dates are a good source of energy and provide a range of nutrients that are important for the health and well-being of pregnant women. However, it is important for pregnant women to be aware of the potential risks of consuming dates, as well as the potential benefits.

One potential risk of consuming dates during pregnancy is the risk of consuming too much sugar. Dates are naturally high in sugar, and consuming large amounts of added sugars during pregnancy can contribute to weight gain and increase the risk of certain health problems. It is important for pregnant women to be mindful of their intake of added sugars and to choose dates in moderation.

In addition, some pregnant women may be allergic to dates or may have sensitivities to them. It is important for pregnant women to be aware of any food allergies or sensitivities they may have and to speak with their healthcare provider if they are concerned about the potential risks of consuming dates.

Overall, dates can be a nutritious and enjoyable part of a healthy diet during pregnancy when consumed in moderation and with appropriate precautions. As with any food, it is important for pregnant women to speak with their healthcare provider about their dietary needs and any potential risks or concerns.

Deli meat

Deli meat, also known as luncheon meat or processed meat, is a type of meat that has been cured, smoked, or otherwise processed and is typically sliced thin and sold in a deli or grocery store. Deli meat includes a variety of products, such as ham, turkey, roast beef, and salami.

During pregnancy, it is generally recommended to avoid or limit the consumption of deli meat. Deli meat is often high in sodium, saturated fat, and other additives, which can increase the risk of certain health problems.

The World Health Organization (WHO) has classified processed meats, including deli meats, as a Group 1 carcinogen, which means that there is sufficient evidence to conclude that they are carcinogenic to humans. The WHO has also classified red meat, including beef, pork, and lamb, as a Group 2A carcinogen, which means that there is limited evidence to suggest that it may be carcinogenic to humans.

Pregnant women who are concerned about the potential health risks of consuming deli meat may want to consider limiting their intake of these products or choosing alternative sources of protein, such as poultry, fish, beans, and legumes.

It is important for pregnant women to speak with their healthcare provider about their dietary needs and any potential risks or concerns. Pregnant women should aim to follow a well-balanced diet that includes a variety of foods from all food groups, including protein-rich foods that are low in saturated fat and additives.

Deviled eggs

Deviled eggs are a type of appetizer or snack food that is made by halving hard-boiled eggs, removing the yolks, and mashing them together with various ingredients, such as mayonnaise, mustard, and spices, before filling the egg whites with the mixture. Deviled eggs are often served chilled or at room temperature.

During pregnancy, it is generally considered safe to consume deviled eggs as part of a healthy diet. Deviled eggs are a good source of protein, which is important for the growth and development of the fetus and for the maintenance of the pregnant woman's tissues. Deviled eggs may also provide other nutrients, such as vitamins and minerals.

However, it is important for pregnant women to be aware of the potential risks of consuming deviled eggs, as well as the potential benefits. Some pregnant women may be allergic to eggs or may have sensitivities to them. In addition, consuming large amounts of deviled eggs may increase the risk of heart disease and other health problems due to their high fat and cholesterol content.

It is generally recommended for pregnant women to consume deviled eggs in moderation and to speak with their healthcare provider if they are concerned about the potential risks of consuming deviled eggs. Pregnant women should also be aware of any food allergies or sensitivities they may have and should speak with their healthcare provider if they are concerned about the potential risks of consuming deviled eggs.

Overall, deviled eggs can be a tasty and convenient part of a healthy diet during pregnancy when consumed in moderation and with appropriate precautions. Pregnant women should speak with their healthcare provider about their dietary needs and any potential risks or concerns.

Dips

Dips are a type of food that is typically made by combining a variety of ingredients, such as spreads, condiments, and seasonings, to create a flavorful sauce or spread that is used for dipping foods, such as chips, crackers, or vegetables. Dips may be made with various types of ingredients, including dairy products, meats, vegetables, and legumes, and may be served hot or cold.

During pregnancy, it is generally considered safe to consume dips as part of a healthy diet. Dips can provide a variety of nutrients, depending on the ingredients used, and may have potential health benefits. However, it is important for pregnant women to be aware of the potential risks of consuming dips, as well as the potential benefits.

Some pregnant women may be allergic to certain ingredients in dips or may have sensitivities to them. In addition, consuming large amounts of dips may increase the risk of weight gain and other health problems due to their high calorie and fat content. Dips may also contain high levels of sodium or other ingredients that may not be suitable for pregnant women who are trying to manage their blood pressure or other health conditions.

It is generally recommended for pregnant women to consume dips in moderation and to speak with their healthcare provider if they are concerned about the potential risks of consuming dips. Pregnant women should also be aware of any food allergies or sensitivities they may have and should speak with their healthcare provider if they are concerned about the potential risks of consuming dips.

Overall, dips can be a flavorful and convenient part of a healthy diet during pregnancy when consumed in moderation and with appropriate precautions. Pregnant women should speak with their healthcare provider about their dietary needs and any potential risks or concerns.

Dried fruit such as apricots and dates

Dried fruit is fruit that has been dehydrated and had most of its water content removed. Dried fruit is a convenient, portable snack that is high in nutrients, including fiber, vitamins, and minerals. Examples of dried fruit include apricots, dates, figs, raisins, and cranberries.

During pregnancy, it is generally considered safe to consume dried fruit in moderation. Dried fruit is a good source of energy and provides a range of nutrients that are important for the health and well-being of pregnant women. However, it is important for pregnant women to be aware of the potential risks of consuming dried fruit, as well as the potential benefits.

One potential risk of consuming dried fruit during pregnancy is the risk of consuming too much sugar. Dried fruit is naturally high in sugar, and consuming large amounts of added sugars during pregnancy can contribute to weight gain and increase the risk of certain health problems. It is important for pregnant women to be mindful of their intake of added sugars and to choose dried fruit in moderation.

In addition, some pregnant women may be allergic to certain types of dried fruit or may have sensitivities to them. It is important for pregnant women to be aware of any food allergies or sensitivities they may have and to speak with their healthcare provider if they are concerned about the potential risks of consuming dried fruit.

Overall, dried fruit can be a nutritious and enjoyable part of a healthy diet during pregnancy when consumed in moderation and with appropriate precautions. As with any food, it is important for pregnant women to speak with their healthcare provider about their dietary needs and any potential risks or concerns.

Dried cranberries

Dried cranberries are a type of fruit that is made by drying cranberries and removing their moisture content. Dried cranberries are often sweetened with sugar or other sweeteners and may be used as a snack or as an ingredient in various types of recipes, such as baked goods or salads.

During pregnancy, it is generally considered safe to consume dried cranberries as part of a healthy diet. Dried cranberries are a good source of nutrients, including vitamins and minerals, and may have potential health benefits. Dried cranberries may also be a good source of antioxidants, which may help to protect the body's cells from damage.

However, it is important for pregnant women to be aware of the potential risks of consuming dried cranberries, as well as the potential benefits. Some pregnant women may be allergic to cranberries or may have sensitivities to them. In addition, consuming large amounts of dried cranberries may increase the risk of weight gain and other health problems due to their high sugar and calorie content.

It is generally recommended for pregnant women to consume dried cranberries in moderation and to speak with their healthcare provider if they are concerned about the potential risks of consuming dried cranberries. Pregnant women should also be aware of any food allergies or sensitivities they may have and should speak with their healthcare provider if they are concerned about the potential risks of consuming dried cranberries.

Overall, dried cranberries can be a tasty and convenient part of a healthy diet during pregnancy when consumed in moderation and with appropriate precautions. Pregnant women should speak with their healthcare provider about their dietary needs and any potential risks or concerns.

Dried mango

Dried mango is a type of fruit that is made by drying mangoes and removing their moisture content. Dried mango is often sweetened with sugar or other sweeteners and may be used as a snack or as an ingredient in various types of recipes, such as baked goods or salads.

During pregnancy, it is generally considered safe to consume dried mango as part of a healthy diet. Dried mango is a good source of nutrients, including vitamins and minerals, and may have potential health benefits. Dried mango may also be a good source of antioxidants, which may help to protect the body's cells from damage.

However, it is important for pregnant women to be aware of the potential risks of consuming dried mango, as well as the potential benefits. Some pregnant women may be allergic to mango or may have sensitivities to it. In addition, consuming large amounts of dried mango may increase the risk of weight gain and other health problems due to its high sugar and calorie content.

It is generally recommended for pregnant women to consume dried mango in moderation and to speak with their healthcare provider if they are concerned about the potential risks of consuming dried mango. Pregnant women should also be aware of any food allergies or sensitivities they may have and should speak with their healthcare provider if they are concerned about the potential risks of consuming dried mango.

Overall, dried mango can be a tasty and convenient part of a healthy diet during pregnancy when consumed in moderation and with appropriate precautions. Pregnant women should speak with their healthcare provider about their dietary needs and any potential risks or concerns.

Dried apricots

Dried apricots are a type of fruit that is made by drying apricots and removing their moisture content. Dried apricots are often sweetened with sugar or other sweeteners and may be used as a snack or as an ingredient in various types of recipes, such as baked goods or salads.

During pregnancy, it is generally considered safe to consume dried apricots as part of a healthy diet. Dried apricots are a good source of nutrients, including vitamins and minerals, and may have potential health benefits. Dried apricots may also be a good source of antioxidants, which may help to protect the body's cells from damage.

However, it is important for pregnant women to be aware of the potential risks of consuming dried apricots, as well as the potential benefits. Some pregnant women may be allergic to apricots or may have sensitivities to them. In addition, consuming large amounts of dried apricots may increase the risk of weight gain and other health problems due to their high sugar and calorie content.

It is generally recommended for pregnant women to consume dried apricots in moderation and to speak with their healthcare provider if they are concerned about the potential risks of consuming dried apricots. Pregnant women should also be aware of any food allergies or sensitivities they may have and should speak with their healthcare provider if they are concerned about the potential risks of consuming dried apricots.

Overall, dried apricots can be a tasty and convenient part of a healthy diet during pregnancy when consumed in moderation and with appropriate precautions. Pregnant women should speak with their healthcare provider about their dietary needs and any potential risks or concerns.

Dried cherries

Dried cherries are a type of fruit that is made by drying cherries and removing their moisture content. Dried cherries are often sweetened with sugar or other sweeteners and may be used as a snack or as an ingredient in various types of recipes, such as baked goods or salads.

During pregnancy, it is generally considered safe to consume dried cherries as part of a healthy diet. Dried cherries are a good source of nutrients, including vitamins and minerals, and may have potential health benefits. Dried cherries may also be a good source of antioxidants, which may help to protect the body's cells from damage.

However, it is important for pregnant women to be aware of the potential risks of consuming dried cherries, as well as the potential benefits. Some pregnant women may be allergic to cherries or may have sensitivities to them. In addition, consuming large amounts of dried cherries may increase the risk of weight gain and other health problems due to their high sugar and calorie content.

It is generally recommended for pregnant women to consume dried cherries in moderation and to speak with their healthcare provider if they are concerned about the potential risks of consuming dried cherries. Pregnant women should also be aware of any food allergies or sensitivities they may have and should speak with their healthcare provider if they are concerned about the potential risks of consuming dried cherries.

Overall, dried cherries can be a tasty and convenient part of a healthy diet during pregnancy when consumed in moderation and with appropriate precautions. Pregnant women should speak with their healthcare provider about their dietary needs and any potential risks or concerns.

Dried pineapples

Dried pineapples are a type of fruit that is made by drying pineapples and removing their moisture content. Dried pineapples are often sweetened with sugar or other sweeteners and may be used as a snack or as an ingredient in various types of recipes, such as baked goods or salads.

During pregnancy, it is generally considered safe to consume dried pineapples as part of a healthy diet. Dried pineapples are a good source of nutrients, including vitamins and minerals, and may have potential health benefits. Dried pineapples may also be a good source of antioxidants, which may help to protect the body's cells from damage.

However, it is important for pregnant women to be aware of the potential risks of consuming dried pineapples, as well as the potential benefits. Some pregnant women may be allergic to pineapples or may have sensitivities to them. In addition, consuming large amounts of dried pineapples may increase the risk of weight gain and other health problems due to their high sugar and calorie content.

It is generally recommended for pregnant women to consume dried pineapples in moderation and to speak with their healthcare provider if they are concerned about the potential risks of consuming dried pineapples. Pregnant women should also be aware of any food allergies or sensitivities they may have and should speak with their healthcare provider if they are concerned about the potential risks of consuming dried pineapples.

Overall, dried pineapples can be a tasty and convenient part of a healthy diet during pregnancy when consumed in moderation and with appropriate precautions. Pregnant women should speak with their healthcare provider about their dietary needs and any potential risks or concerns.

Dried prunes

Dried prunes are a type of fruit that is made by drying plums and removing their moisture content. Dried prunes are often sweetened with sugar or other sweeteners and may be used as a snack or as an ingredient in various types of recipes, such as baked goods or salads.

During pregnancy, it is generally considered safe to consume dried prunes as part of a healthy diet. Dried prunes are a good source of nutrients, including vitamins and minerals, and may have potential health benefits. Dried prunes may also be a good source of antioxidants, which may help to protect the body's cells from damage.

However, it is important for pregnant women to be aware of the potential risks of consuming dried prunes, as well as the potential benefits. Some pregnant women may be allergic to prunes or may have sensitivities to them. In addition, consuming large amounts of dried prunes may increase the risk of weight gain and other health problems due to their high sugar and calorie content.

It is generally recommended for pregnant women to consume dried prunes in moderation and to speak with their healthcare provider if they are concerned about the potential risks of consuming dried prunes. Pregnant women should also be aware of any food allergies or sensitivities they may have and should speak with their healthcare provider if they are concerned about the potential risks of consuming dried prunes.

Overall, dried prunes can be a tasty and convenient part of a healthy diet during pregnancy when consumed in moderation and with appropriate precautions. Pregnant women should speak with their healthcare provider about their dietary needs and any potential risks or concerns.

Dried raisins

Dried raisins are a type of fruit that is made by drying grapes and removing their moisture content. Dried raisins are often sweetened with sugar or other sweeteners and may be used as a snack or as an ingredient in various types of recipes, such as baked goods or salads.

During pregnancy, it is generally considered safe to consume dried raisins as part of a healthy diet. Dried raisins are a good source of nutrients, including vitamins and minerals, and may have potential health benefits. Dried raisins may also be a good source of antioxidants, which may help to protect the body's cells from damage.

However, it is important for pregnant women to be aware of the potential risks of consuming dried raisins, as well as the potential benefits. Some pregnant women may be allergic to raisins or may have sensitivities to them. In addition, consuming large amounts of dried raisins may increase the risk of weight gain and other health problems due to their high sugar and calorie content.

It is generally recommended for pregnant women to consume dried raisins in moderation and to speak with their healthcare provider if they are concerned about the potential risks of consuming dried raisins. Pregnant women should also be aware of any food allergies or sensitivities they may have and should speak with their healthcare provider if they are concerned about the potential risks of consuming dried raisins.

Overall, dried raisins can be a tasty and convenient part of a healthy diet during pregnancy when consumed in moderation and with appropriate precautions. Pregnant women should speak with their healthcare provider about their dietary needs and any potential risks or concerns.

Dried apples

Dried apples are a type of fruit that is made by drying apples and removing their moisture content. Dried apples are often sweetened with sugar or other sweeteners and may be used as a snack or as an ingredient in various types of recipes, such as baked goods or salads.

During pregnancy, it is generally considered safe to consume dried apples as part of a healthy diet. Dried apples are a good source of nutrients, including vitamins and minerals, and may have potential health benefits. Dried apples may also be a good source of antioxidants, which may help to protect the body's cells from damage.

However, it is important for pregnant women to be aware of the potential risks of consuming dried apples, as well as the potential benefits. Some pregnant women may be allergic to apples or may have sensitivities to them. In addition, consuming large amounts of dried apples may increase the risk of weight gain and other health problems due to their high sugar and calorie content.

It is generally recommended for pregnant women to consume dried apples in moderation and to speak with their healthcare provider if they are concerned about the potential risks of consuming dried apples. Pregnant women should also be aware of any food allergies or sensitivities they may have and should speak with their healthcare provider if they are concerned about the potential risks of consuming dried apples.

Overall, dried apples can be a tasty and convenient part of a healthy diet during pregnancy when consumed in moderation and with appropriate precautions. Pregnant women should speak with

their healthcare provider about their dietary needs and any potential risks or concerns.

Dried blueberries

Dried blueberries are a type of fruit that is made by drying blueberries and removing their moisture content. Dried blueberries are often sweetened with sugar or other sweeteners and may be used as a snack or as an ingredient in various types of recipes, such as baked goods or salads.

During pregnancy, it is generally considered safe to consume dried blueberries as part of a healthy diet. Dried blueberries are a good source of nutrients, including vitamins and minerals, and may have potential health benefits. Dried blueberries may also be a good source of antioxidants, which may help to protect the body's cells from damage.

However, it is important for pregnant women to be aware of the potential risks of consuming dried blueberries, as well as the potential benefits. Some pregnant women may be allergic to blueberries or may have sensitivities to them. In addition, consuming large amounts of dried blueberries may increase the risk of weight gain and other health problems due to their high sugar and calorie content.

It is generally recommended for pregnant women to consume dried blueberries in moderation and to speak with their healthcare provider if they are concerned about the potential risks of consuming dried blueberries. Pregnant women should also be aware of any food allergies or sensitivities they may have and should speak with their healthcare provider if they are concerned about the potential risks of consuming dried blueberries.

Overall, dried blueberries can be a tasty and convenient part of a healthy diet during pregnancy when consumed in moderation and with appropriate precautions. Pregnant women should speak with

their healthcare provider about their dietary needs and any potential risks or concerns.

Dried peaches

Dried peaches are a type of fruit that is made by drying peaches and removing their moisture content. Dried peaches are often sweetened with sugar or other sweeteners and may be used as a snack or as an ingredient in various types of recipes, such as baked goods or salads.

During pregnancy, it is generally considered safe to consume dried peaches as part of a healthy diet. Dried peaches are a good source of nutrients, including vitamins and minerals, and may have potential health benefits. Dried peaches may also be a good source of antioxidants, which may help to protect the body's cells from damage.

However, it is important for pregnant women to be aware of the potential risks of consuming dried peaches, as well as the potential benefits. Some pregnant women may be allergic to peaches or may have sensitivities to them. In addition, consuming large amounts of dried peaches may increase the risk of weight gain and other health problems due to their high sugar and calorie content.

It is generally recommended for pregnant women to consume dried peaches in moderation and to speak with their healthcare provider if they are concerned about the potential risks of consuming dried peaches. Pregnant women should also be aware of any food allergies or sensitivities they may have and should speak with their healthcare provider if they are concerned about the potential risks of consuming dried peaches.

Overall, dried peaches can be a tasty and convenient part of a healthy diet during pregnancy when consumed in moderation and with appropriate precautions. Pregnant women should speak with their healthcare provider about their dietary needs and any potential risks or concerns.

Dried pears

Dried pears are a type of fruit that is made by drying pears and removing their moisture content. Dried pears are often sweetened with sugar or other sweeteners and may be used as a snack or as an ingredient in various types of recipes, such as baked goods or salads.

During pregnancy, it is generally considered safe to consume dried pears as part of a healthy diet. Dried pears are a good source of nutrients, including vitamins and minerals, and may have potential health benefits. Dried pears may also be a good source of antioxidants, which may help to protect the body's cells from damage.

However, it is important for pregnant women to be aware of the potential risks of consuming dried pears, as well as the potential benefits. Some pregnant women may be allergic to pears or may have sensitivities to them. In addition, consuming large amounts of dried pears may increase the risk of weight gain and other health problems due to their high sugar and calorie content.

It is generally recommended for pregnant women to consume dried pears in moderation and to speak with their healthcare provider if they are concerned about the potential risks of consuming dried pears. Pregnant women should also be aware of any food allergies or sensitivities they may have and should speak with their healthcare provider if they are concerned about the potential risks of consuming dried pears.

Overall, dried pears can be a tasty and convenient part of a healthy diet during pregnancy when consumed in moderation and with appropriate precautions. Pregnant women should speak with their healthcare provider about their dietary needs and any potential risks or concerns.

Dried plums

Dried plums, also known as prunes, are a type of fruit that is made by drying plums and removing their moisture content. Dried plums are often sweetened with sugar or other sweeteners and may be used as a snack or as an ingredient in various types of recipes, such as baked goods or salads.

During pregnancy, it is generally considered safe to consume dried plums as part of a healthy diet. Dried plums are a good source of nutrients, including vitamins and minerals, and may have potential health benefits. Dried plums may also be a good source of antioxidants, which may help to protect the body's cells from damage.

However, it is important for pregnant women to be aware of the potential risks of consuming dried plums, as well as the potential benefits. Some pregnant women may be allergic to plums or may have sensitivities to them. In addition, consuming large amounts of dried plums may increase the risk of weight gain and other health problems due to their high sugar and calorie content.

It is generally recommended for pregnant women to consume dried plums in moderation and to speak with their healthcare provider if they are concerned about the potential risks of consuming dried plums. Pregnant women should also be aware of any food allergies or sensitivities they may have and should speak with their healthcare provider if they are concerned about the potential risks of consuming dried plums.

Overall, dried plums can be a tasty and convenient part of a healthy diet during pregnancy when consumed in moderation and with appropriate precautions. Pregnant women should speak with their healthcare provider about their dietary needs and any potential risks or concerns.

Dried strawberries

Dried strawberries are a type of fruit that is made by drying strawberries and removing their moisture content. Dried strawberries are often sweetened with sugar or other sweeteners and may be used as a snack or as an ingredient in various types of recipes, such as baked goods or salads.

During pregnancy, it is generally considered safe to consume dried strawberries as part of a healthy diet. Dried strawberries are a good source of nutrients, including vitamins and minerals, and may have potential health benefits. Dried strawberries may also be a good source of antioxidants, which may help to protect the body's cells from damage.

However, it is important for pregnant women to be aware of the potential risks of consuming dried strawberries, as well as the potential benefits. Some pregnant women may be allergic to strawberries or may have sensitivities to them. In addition, consuming large amounts of dried strawberries may increase the risk of weight gain and other health problems due to their high sugar and calorie content.

It is generally recommended for pregnant women to consume dried strawberries in moderation and to speak with their healthcare provider if they are concerned about the potential risks of consuming dried strawberries. Pregnant women should also be aware of any food allergies or sensitivities they may have and should speak with their healthcare provider if they are concerned about the potential risks of consuming dried strawberries.

Overall, dried strawberries can be a tasty and convenient part of a healthy diet during pregnancy when consumed in moderation and with appropriate precautions. Pregnant women should speak with their healthcare provider about their dietary needs and any potential risks or concerns.

Dried tomatoes

Dried tomatoes are a type of fruit that is made by drying tomatoes and removing their moisture content. Dried tomatoes are often sweetened with sugar or other sweeteners and may be used as a snack or as an ingredient in various types of recipes, such as baked goods or salads.

During pregnancy, it is generally considered safe to consume dried tomatoes as part of a healthy diet. Dried tomatoes are a good source of nutrients, including vitamins and minerals, and may have potential health benefits. Dried tomatoes may also be a good source of antioxidants, which may help to protect the body's cells from damage.

However, it is important for pregnant women to be aware of the potential risks of consuming dried tomatoes, as well as the potential benefits. Some pregnant women may be allergic to tomatoes or may have sensitivities to them. In addition, consuming large amounts of dried tomatoes may increase the risk of weight gain and other health problems due to their high sugar and calorie content.

It is generally recommended for pregnant women to consume dried tomatoes in moderation and to speak with their healthcare provider if they are concerned about the potential risks of consuming dried tomatoes. Pregnant women should also be aware of any food allergies or sensitivities they may have and should speak with their healthcare provider if they are concerned about the potential risks of consuming dried tomatoes.

Overall, dried tomatoes can be a tasty and convenient part of a healthy diet during pregnancy when consumed in moderation and with appropriate precautions. Pregnant women should speak with their healthcare provider about their dietary needs and any potential risks or concerns.

Dried tropical fruit

Dried tropical fruit is a type of fruit that is made by drying fruit from tropical regions, such as the Caribbean, Central America, and South America, and removing their moisture content. Dried tropical fruit is often sweetened with sugar or other sweeteners and may be used as a snack or as an ingredient in various types of recipes, such as baked goods or salads.

During pregnancy, it is generally considered safe to consume dried tropical fruit as part of a healthy diet. Dried tropical fruit is a good source of nutrients, including vitamins and minerals, and may have potential health benefits. Dried tropical fruit may also be a good source of antioxidants, which may help to protect the body's cells from damage.

However, it is important for pregnant women to be aware of the potential risks of consuming dried tropical fruit, as well as the potential benefits. Some pregnant women may be allergic to certain types of tropical fruit or may have sensitivities to them. In addition, consuming large amounts of dried tropical fruit may increase the risk of weight gain and other health problems due to their high sugar and calorie content.

It is generally recommended for pregnant women to consume dried tropical fruit in moderation and to speak with their healthcare provider if they are concerned about the potential risks of consuming dried tropical fruit. Pregnant women should also be aware of any food allergies or sensitivities they may have and should speak with their healthcare provider if they are concerned about the potential risks of consuming dried tropical fruit.

Overall, dried tropical fruit can be a tasty and convenient part of a healthy diet during pregnancy when consumed in moderation and with appropriate precautions. Pregnant women should speak with their healthcare provider about their dietary needs and any potential risks or concerns.

Dried tuna

Dried tuna is a type of fish that is made by drying tuna and removing its moisture content. Dried tuna is often salted or flavored and may be used as a snack or as an ingredient in various types of recipes, such as soups or stews.

During pregnancy, it is generally considered safe to consume dried tuna as part of a healthy diet in moderation. Tuna is a good source of protein, omega-3 fatty acids, and other nutrients that are important for fetal development and the health of the mother. However, it is important for pregnant women to be aware of the potential risks of consuming dried tuna, as well as the potential benefits.

One potential risk of consuming dried tuna during pregnancy is the risk of mercury exposure. Some types of tuna, such as albacore and tuna steaks, may contain higher levels of mercury than others, such as canned light tuna. Pregnant women should be aware of the types of tuna they are consuming and should follow guidelines for safe consumption to minimize the risk of mercury exposure.

In addition, pregnant women should be aware of the potential risks of consuming large amounts of dried tuna due to its high sodium content. Consuming large amounts of sodium may increase the risk of high blood pressure and other health problems during pregnancy.

It is generally recommended for pregnant women to consume dried tuna in moderation and to speak with their healthcare provider if they are concerned about the potential risks of consuming dried tuna. Pregnant women should also be aware of any food allergies or sensitivities they may have and should speak with their healthcare provider if they are concerned about the potential risks of consuming dried tuna.

Overall, dried tuna can be a tasty and convenient part of a healthy diet during pregnancy when consumed in moderation and with appropriate precautions. Pregnant women should speak with their healthcare provider about their dietary needs and any potential risks or concerns.

Donuts

Donuts are a type of sweet, deep-fried pastry that is often shaped like a ring and is typically topped with frosting, sprinkles, or other types of decorations. Donuts may be flavored with various ingredients, such as chocolate, fruit, or spices.

During pregnancy, it is generally considered safe to consume donuts as part of a healthy diet. Donuts are a good source of carbohydrates, which provide energy to the body, and may have potential health benefits. However, it is important for pregnant women to be aware of the potential risks of consuming donuts, as well as the potential benefits.

Some pregnant women may be allergic to donuts or may have sensitivities to them. In addition, consuming large amounts of donuts may increase the risk of weight gain and other health problems due to their high calorie, fat, and sugar content. Donuts may also contain high levels of sodium or other ingredients that may not be suitable for pregnant women who are trying to manage their blood pressure or other health conditions.

It is generally recommended for pregnant women to consume donuts in moderation and to speak with their healthcare provider if they are concerned about the potential risks of consuming donuts. Pregnant women should also be aware of any food allergies or sensitivities they may have and should speak with their healthcare provider if they are concerned about the potential risks of consuming donuts.

Overall, donuts can be a tasty and convenient part of a healthy diet during pregnancy when consumed in moderation and with appropriate precautions. Pregnant women should speak with their healthcare provider about their dietary needs and any potential risks or concerns.

Eggplant

Eggplant is a type of vegetable that is native to South Asia and is widely cultivated for its edible fruit. Eggplant is a good source of nutrients, including fiber, potassium, and antioxidants. Eggplant is available in a variety of shapes, sizes, and colors, and is often used in a variety of dishes, including stir-fries, grilled dishes, and baked goods.

During pregnancy, it is generally considered safe to consume eggplant in moderation. Eggplant is a good source of nutrients that are important for the health and well-being of pregnant women. However, it is important for pregnant women to be aware of the potential risks of consuming eggplant, as well as the potential benefits.

One potential risk of consuming eggplant during pregnancy is the risk of consuming too much solanine, a toxic compound that is present in some plants, including eggplant. Solanine can cause symptoms such as nausea, vomiting, and diarrhea if consumed in large amounts. However, solanine is generally only found in the leaves and stems of eggplant plants, and the fruit of the eggplant plant is generally considered safe to consume.

In addition, some pregnant women may be allergic to eggplant or may have sensitivities to it. It is important for pregnant women to be aware of any food allergies or sensitivities they may have and to speak with their healthcare provider if they are concerned about the potential risks of consuming eggplant.

Overall, eggplant can be a nutritious and enjoyable part of a healthy diet during pregnancy when consumed in moderation and with appropriate precautions. As with any food, it is important for pregnant women to speak with their healthcare provider about their dietary needs and any potential risks or concerns.

Eggnog

Eggnog is a creamy, sweet beverage that is traditionally made with milk, cream, sugar, and eggs, and often flavored with spices such as cinnamon and nutmeg. Eggnog is often served during the holiday season.

During pregnancy, it is generally considered safe to consume small amounts of eggnog as part of a healthy diet. However, it is important for pregnant women to be aware of the potential risks of consuming eggnog, as well as the potential benefits.

One potential risk of consuming eggnog during pregnancy is the risk of food poisoning due to the raw eggs used in the recipe. Raw eggs may contain bacteria such as Salmonella, which can cause food poisoning. To minimize the risk of food poisoning, pregnant women should ensure that the eggnog they are consuming has been made with pasteurized eggs or that the eggs have been cooked to a safe temperature.

In addition, pregnant women should be aware of the potential risks of consuming large amounts of eggnog due to its high sugar and calorie content. Consuming large amounts of sugar and calories may increase the risk of weight gain and other health problems during pregnancy.

It is generally recommended for pregnant women to consume eggnog in moderation and to speak with their healthcare provider if they are concerned about the potential risks of consuming eggnog. Pregnant women should also be aware of any food allergies or sensitivities they may have and should speak with their healthcare provider if they are concerned about the potential risks of consuming eggnog.

Overall, eggnog can be a tasty and convenient part of a healthy diet during pregnancy when consumed in moderation and with appropriate precautions. Pregnant women should speak with their healthcare provider about their dietary needs and any potential risks or concerns.

Eggs

It is generally recommended that pregnant women avoid consuming raw or partially cooked eggs. This is because raw or partially cooked eggs can contain harmful bacteria that can cause foodborne illness.

Pregnant women are at increased risk of foodborne illness because their immune systems are compromised during pregnancy. Consuming contaminated raw or partially cooked eggs can increase the risk of contracting a bacterial infection, such as salmonella. This infection can cause serious complications, including miscarriage, stillbirth, and severe illness in the mother.

To reduce the risk of foodborne illness, it is important for pregnant women to follow safe food handling practices, including washing their hands thoroughly with soap and water before handling food and cooking eggs to a safe internal temperature. Pregnant women should also be cautious about consuming other types of raw or undercooked products, such as raw sprouts, uncooked or undercooked meats, poultry, seafood, and eggs, and unpasteurized milk and dairy products.

In summary, it is generally recommended that pregnant women avoid consuming raw or partially cooked eggs to reduce the risk of contracting a bacterial infection. Pregnant women should follow safe food handling practices and be cautious about consuming other types of raw or undercooked products.

Edamame

Edamame is a type of food that is made from young, green soybeans that are cooked and often salted. Edamame is a popular snack in East Asia and is increasingly being consumed in other parts of the world. Edamame is a good source of protein, fiber, and nutrients, such as iron and calcium.

During pregnancy, it is generally considered safe to consume edamame in moderation. Edamame is a good source of nutrients that are important for the health and well-being of pregnant women. However, it is important for pregnant women to be aware of the potential risks of consuming edamame, as well as the potential benefits.

One potential risk of consuming edamame during pregnancy is the risk of consuming too much soy. Some studies have suggested that consuming large amounts of soy during pregnancy may have negative effects on fetal development, although the evidence on this topic is mixed. It is important for pregnant women to be mindful of their intake of soy and to choose edamame in moderation.

In addition, some pregnant women may be allergic to soy or may have sensitivities to it. It is important for pregnant women to be aware of any food allergies or sensitivities they may have and to speak with their healthcare provider if they are concerned about the potential risks of consuming edamame.

Overall, edamame can be a nutritious and enjoyable part of a healthy diet during pregnancy when consumed in moderation and with appropriate precautions. As with any food, it is important for pregnant women to speak with their healthcare provider about their dietary needs and any potential risks or concerns.

Energy drinks

Energy drinks are beverages that are marketed as providing a boost of energy, typically through the use of caffeine and other stimulant ingredients. Energy drinks are often consumed by people who are looking to increase their energy levels or improve their physical or mental performance.

During pregnancy, it is generally recommended to avoid or limit the consumption of energy drinks. Energy drinks are high in caffeine and other stimulant ingredients, which can have negative effects on the body, particularly in large amounts.

The American College of Obstetricians and Gynecologists (ACOG) recommends that pregnant women limit their caffeine intake to 200 milligrams per day, which is equivalent to about one 12-ounce cup of coffee. Energy drinks can contain significantly more caffeine than this amount, and consuming large amounts of caffeine during pregnancy can increase the risk of certain health problems, such as miscarriage, preterm birth, and low birth weight.

In addition, energy drinks may contain other ingredients, such as sugar and artificial sweeteners, that can have negative effects on the body when consumed in large amounts. It is important for pregnant women to be mindful of the ingredients in energy drinks and to choose alternative sources of hydration and energy, such as water and other low-caffeine beverages.

Overall, energy drinks should be avoided or consumed in moderation during pregnancy due to the potential risks associated with their high caffeine and other stimulant content. Pregnant women should speak with their healthcare provider about their dietary needs and any potential risks or concerns.

Enchiladas

Enchiladas are a type of Mexican dish that consists of corn tortillas filled with a variety of ingredients, such as meat, cheese, beans, and vegetables, and then rolled and baked or fried. The filled tortillas are often covered with a sauce, such as a tomato or mole sauce, and topped with additional cheese or other toppings.

During pregnancy, it is generally considered safe to consume enchiladas as part of a healthy diet in moderation. Enchiladas can be a good source of protein, vitamins, and minerals, and may have potential health benefits when consumed as part of a balanced diet.

However, it is important for pregnant women to be aware of the potential risks of consuming enchiladas, as well as the potential benefits. Some pregnant women may be allergic to certain ingredients used in enchiladas or may have sensitivities to them. In addition, consuming large amounts of enchiladas may increase the risk of weight gain and other health problems due to their high calorie and fat content.

It is generally recommended for pregnant women to consume enchiladas in moderation and to speak with their healthcare provider if they are concerned about the potential risks of consuming enchiladas. Pregnant women should also be aware of any food allergies or sensitivities they may have and should speak with their healthcare provider if they are concerned about the potential risks of consuming enchiladas.

Overall, enchiladas can be a tasty and convenient part of a healthy diet during pregnancy when consumed in moderation and with appropriate precautions. Pregnant women should speak with their healthcare provider about their dietary needs and any potential risks or concerns.

Exercise

Exercise is an important part of maintaining a healthy pregnancy and can have a range of benefits for both the mother and the developing baby. Exercise can help to improve cardiovascular health, manage stress, and control weight gain during pregnancy.

However, it is important for pregnant women to be mindful of their exercise habits and to speak with their healthcare provider before starting or continuing an exercise program during pregnancy. Pregnancy is a time of physical and hormonal changes, and it is important for pregnant women to listen to their bodies and adjust their exercise habits accordingly.

Pregnant women should aim to engage in moderate-intensity aerobic exercise, such as brisk walking or swimming, for at least 150 minutes per week. However, it is important for pregnant women to speak with their healthcare provider about their specific exercise needs and any potential risks or concerns.

There are some types of exercise that may be inappropriate or risky for pregnant women, such as activities that involve high impact or contact, or activities that have a high risk of falling or injury. Pregnant women should avoid these types of activities and choose alternatives that are safer and more appropriate for their physical abilities.

Overall, exercise is an important part of a healthy pregnancy, and pregnant women should aim to engage in regular physical activity that is appropriate for their fitness level and individual needs. However, it is important for pregnant women to speak with their healthcare provider before starting or continuing an exercise program during pregnancy.

Fast food

Fast food is a type of food that is typically prepared and served quickly, often at a fast food restaurant or drive-thru. Fast food is often high in calories, saturated fat, and sodium, and can contribute to weight gain and an increased risk of certain health problems.

During pregnancy, it is generally recommended to avoid or limit the consumption of fast food. Pregnancy is a time of physical and hormonal changes, and it is important for pregnant women to pay attention to their diet and to choose foods that are nutritious and supportive of their health and the health of their developing baby.

Fast food is often high in calories, saturated fat, and sodium, and can contribute to weight gain and an increased risk of certain health problems, such as high blood pressure, diabetes, and heart disease. Pregnant women who consume large amounts of fast food may be at increased risk of these health problems, as well as other negative health outcomes.

In addition, fast food may contain additives and preservatives that can be harmful to pregnant women and their developing babies. Pregnant women should aim to choose foods that are minimally processed and free of additives and preservatives, whenever possible.

Overall, fast food should be avoided or consumed in moderation during pregnancy due to the potential risks associated with its high calorie, fat, and sodium content, as well as the potential presence of additives and preservatives. Pregnant women should aim to follow a well-balanced diet that includes a variety of foods from all food groups, and should speak with their healthcare provider about their dietary needs and any potential risks or concerns.

Fajita seasoning

Fajita seasoning is a blend of spices that is typically used to flavor fajitas, which are a type of Mexican dish made with grilled or sautéed slices of meat, vegetables, and spices, served on a tortilla or over rice. Fajita seasoning may include a combination of herbs and spices such as chili powder, cumin, paprika, garlic, and onion.

During pregnancy, it is generally considered safe to consume fajita seasoning as part of a healthy diet in moderation. Fajita seasoning can add flavor and nutrition to a variety of dishes, and may have potential health benefits when consumed as part of a balanced diet.

However, it is important for pregnant women to be aware of the potential risks of consuming fajita seasoning, as well as the potential benefits. Some pregnant women may be allergic to certain ingredients used in fajita seasoning or may have sensitivities to them. In addition, consuming large amounts of fajita seasoning may increase the risk of certain health problems due to the high levels of certain ingredients, such as sodium or certain spices.

It is generally recommended for pregnant women to consume fajita seasoning in moderation and to speak with their healthcare provider if they are concerned about the potential risks of consuming fajita seasoning. Pregnant women should also be aware of any food allergies or sensitivities they may have and should speak with their healthcare provider if they are concerned about the potential risks of consuming fajita seasoning.

Overall, fajita seasoning can be a convenient and flavorful addition to a healthy diet during pregnancy when consumed in moderation and with appropriate precautions. Pregnant women should speak with their healthcare provider about their dietary needs and any potential risks or concerns.

Falafel

Falafel is a traditional Middle Eastern dish made from ground chickpeas or other legumes, mixed with herbs and spices, and then shaped into balls or patties and deep-fried. Falafel is often served in pita bread or as a topping for salads and other dishes.

During pregnancy, it is generally considered safe to consume falafel as part of a healthy diet in moderation. Falafel can be a good source of protein, fiber, and other nutrients, and may have potential health benefits when consumed as part of a balanced diet.

However, it is important for pregnant women to be aware of the potential risks of consuming falafel, as well as the potential benefits. Some pregnant women may be allergic to legumes, such as chickpeas, or may have sensitivities to them. In addition, consuming large amounts of falafel may increase the risk of weight gain and other health problems due to their high calorie and fat content.

It is generally recommended for pregnant women to consume falafel in moderation and to speak with their healthcare provider if they are concerned about the potential risks of consuming falafel. Pregnant women should also be aware of any food allergies or sensitivities they may have and should speak with their healthcare provider if they are concerned about the potential risks of consuming falafel.

Overall, falafel can be a tasty and convenient part of a healthy diet during pregnancy when consumed in moderation and with appropriate precautions. Pregnant women should speak with their healthcare provider about their dietary needs and any potential risks or concerns.

Feta cheese

Feta cheese is a type of cheese that is traditionally made from sheep's milk or a combination of sheep's and goat's milk. It is a crumbly, salty cheese with a tangy flavor that is often used in salads, sandwiches, and other dishes.

During pregnancy, it is generally considered safe to consume feta cheese as part of a healthy diet in moderation. Feta cheese can be a good source of protein, calcium, and other nutrients, and may have potential health benefits when consumed as part of a balanced diet.

However, it is important for pregnant women to be aware of the potential risks of consuming feta cheese, as well as the potential benefits. Some pregnant women may be allergic to dairy products or may have sensitivities to them. In addition, consuming large amounts of feta cheese may increase the risk of weight gain and other health problems due to its high calorie and fat content.

It is generally recommended for pregnant women to consume feta cheese in moderation and to speak with their healthcare provider if they are concerned about the potential risks of consuming feta cheese. Pregnant women should also be aware of any food allergies or sensitivities they may have and should speak with their healthcare provider if they are concerned about the potential risks of consuming feta cheese.

Overall, feta cheese can be a tasty and convenient part of a healthy diet during pregnancy when consumed in moderation and with appropriate precautions. Pregnant women should speak with their healthcare provider about their dietary needs and any potential risks or concerns.

Filet mignon

Filet mignon is a type of beef steak that is cut from the tenderloin, a lean and tender muscle located near the rear of the cow. It is typically a small, thick cut of meat that is known for its delicate flavor and texture. Filet mignon is often served as a high-end dish in restaurants and is often prepared by grilling, pan-frying, or roasting.

During pregnancy, it is generally considered safe to consume filet mignon as part of a healthy diet in moderation. Filet mignon can be a good source of protein, iron, and other nutrients, and may have potential health benefits when consumed as part of a balanced diet.

However, it is important for pregnant women to be aware of the potential risks of consuming filet mignon, as well as the potential benefits. Some pregnant women may be allergic to certain types of meat or may have sensitivities to them. In addition, consuming large amounts of filet mignon may increase the risk of weight gain and other health problems due to its high calorie and fat content.

It is generally recommended for pregnant women to consume filet mignon in moderation and to speak with their healthcare provider if they are concerned about the potential risks of consuming filet mignon. Pregnant women should also be aware of any food allergies or sensitivities they may have and should speak with their healthcare provider if they are concerned about the potential risks of consuming filet mignon.

Overall, filet mignon can be a tasty and convenient part of a healthy diet during pregnancy when consumed in moderation and with appropriate precautions. Pregnant women should speak with their healthcare provider about their dietary needs and any potential risks or concerns.

Fish

It is generally recommended that pregnant women avoid consuming high-mercury fish, such as shark, swordfish, king mackerel, and tilefish. This is because these types of fish can contain high levels of mercury, which can be harmful to the developing fetus.

Mercury is a toxic metal that can accumulate in the body over time. When pregnant women consume high levels of mercury, it can pass through the placenta and reach the developing fetus, potentially causing harm. Mercury can affect the developing brain and nervous system, leading to developmental delays, learning problems, and other long-term health effects.

The Food and Drug Administration (FDA) and the Environmental Protection Agency (EPA) have issued guidelines for pregnant women and women who may become pregnant, breastfeeding women, and young children to limit their consumption of certain types of fish that are high in mercury. These types of fish include shark, swordfish, king mackerel, and tilefish, as well as some types of tuna.

Pregnant women can still include fish in their diet, but it is important to choose low-mercury options. Good choices include salmon, pollock, catfish, and shrimp. It is also recommended that pregnant women limit their consumption of albacore tuna to no more than 6 ounces per week.

In summary, it is generally recommended that pregnant women avoid consuming high-mercury fish, such as shark, swordfish, king mackerel, and tilefish, to reduce the risk of exposing the developing fetus to harmful levels of mercury. Pregnant women can still include fish in their diet, but it is important to choose low-mercury options and to limit their consumption of albacore tuna.

Fish sticks

Fish sticks, also known as fish fingers, are a popular food item that consists of small, breaded and fried pieces of fish. They are often served as a snack or as part of a meal and are typically made from whitefish, such as cod or haddock.

During pregnancy, it is generally considered safe to consume fish sticks as part of a healthy diet in moderation. Fish sticks can be a good source of protein, omega-3 fatty acids, and other nutrients, and may have potential health benefits when consumed as part of a balanced diet.

However, it is important for pregnant women to be aware of the potential risks of consuming fish sticks, as well as the potential benefits. Some pregnant women may be allergic to certain types of fish or may have sensitivities to them. In addition, consuming large amounts of fish sticks may increase the risk of weight gain and other health problems due to their high calorie and fat content.

It is generally recommended for pregnant women to consume fish sticks in moderation and to speak with their healthcare provider if they are concerned about the potential risks of consuming fish sticks. Pregnant women should also be aware of any food allergies or sensitivities they may have and should speak with their healthcare provider if they are concerned about the potential risks of consuming fish sticks.

Overall, fish sticks can be a tasty and convenient part of a healthy diet during pregnancy when consumed in moderation and with appropriate precautions. Pregnant women should speak with their healthcare provider about their dietary needs and any potential risks or concerns.

Flatbread

Flatbread is a type of bread that is thin and typically made from flour, water, and other ingredients such as yeast or baking powder. It is often baked in an oven or cooked on a stovetop and can be served as a snack or as part of a meal. Flatbread can come in a variety of shapes and sizes, and can be made from a variety of grains including wheat, corn, and rice.

During pregnancy, it is generally considered safe to consume flatbread as part of a healthy diet in moderation. Flatbread can be a good source of complex carbohydrates, fiber, and other nutrients, and may have potential health benefits when consumed as part of a balanced diet.

However, it is important for pregnant women to be aware of the potential risks of consuming flatbread, as well as the potential benefits. Some pregnant women may be allergic to certain types of grains or may have sensitivities to them. In addition, consuming large amounts of flatbread may increase the risk of weight gain and other health problems due to its high calorie and carbohydrate content.

It is generally recommended for pregnant women to consume flatbread in moderation and to speak with their healthcare provider if they are concerned about the potential risks of consuming flatbread. Pregnant women should also be aware of any food allergies or sensitivities they may have and should speak with their healthcare provider if they are concerned about the potential risks of consuming flatbread.

Overall, flatbread can be a tasty and convenient part of a healthy diet during pregnancy when consumed in moderation and with appropriate precautions. Pregnant women should speak with their healthcare provider about their dietary needs and any potential risks or concerns.

Flounder

Flounder is a type of fish that belongs to the flatfish family. It is known for its flat, oval-shaped body and has a delicate, mild flavor. Flounder is often served as a high-end dish in restaurants and is often prepared by grilling, pan-frying, or baking.

During pregnancy, it is generally considered safe to consume flounder as part of a healthy diet in moderation. Flounder can be a good source of protein, omega-3 fatty acids, and other nutrients, and may have potential health benefits when consumed as part of a balanced diet.

However, it is important for pregnant women to be aware of the potential risks of consuming flounder, as well as the potential benefits. Some pregnant women may be allergic to certain types of fish or may have sensitivities to them. In addition, consuming large amounts of flounder may increase the risk of weight gain and other health problems due to its high calorie and fat content.

It is generally recommended for pregnant women to consume flounder in moderation and to speak with their healthcare provider if they are concerned about the potential risks of consuming flounder. Pregnant women should also be aware of any food allergies or sensitivities they may have and should speak with their healthcare provider if they are concerned about the potential risks of consuming flounder.

Overall, flounder can be a tasty and convenient part of a healthy diet during pregnancy when consumed in moderation and with appropriate precautions. Pregnant women should speak with their healthcare provider about their dietary needs and any potential risks or concerns.

French fries

French fries, also known as chips or fried potatoes, are a popular food item that consists of thin, fried slices of potatoes. They are often served as a snack or as part of a meal and are typically seasoned with salt and other spices. French fries can be cooked at home or purchased at restaurants, fast food chains, and other food establishments.

During pregnancy, it is generally considered safe to consume French fries in moderation as part of a healthy diet. However, it is important for pregnant women to be aware of the potential risks of consuming French fries, as well as the potential benefits.

Some pregnant women may be allergic to potatoes or may have sensitivities to them. In addition, consuming large amounts of French fries may increase the risk of weight gain and other health problems due to their high calorie, fat, and salt content. French fries are also often fried in oil, which can contribute to an unhealthy diet if consumed in large amounts.

It is generally recommended for pregnant women to consume French fries in moderation and to speak with their healthcare provider if they are concerned about the potential risks of consuming French fries. Pregnant women should also be aware of any food allergies or sensitivities they may have and should speak with their healthcare provider if they are concerned about the potential risks of consuming French fries.

Overall, French fries can be a tasty and convenient part of a healthy diet during pregnancy when consumed in moderation and with appropriate precautions. Pregnant women should speak with

their healthcare provider about their dietary needs and any potential risks or concerns.

Fried catfish

Fried catfish is a type of fish that is often served as a high-end dish in restaurants and is often prepared by frying thin slices of catfish in a mixture of flour and spices. Catfish is known for its flaky, white flesh and has a delicate, mild flavor.

During pregnancy, it is generally considered safe to consume fried catfish as part of a healthy diet in moderation. Fried catfish can be a good source of protein, omega-3 fatty acids, and other nutrients, and may have potential health benefits when consumed as part of a balanced diet.

However, it is important for pregnant women to be aware of the potential risks of consuming fried catfish, as well as the potential benefits. Some pregnant women may be allergic to certain types of fish or may have sensitivities to them. In addition, consuming large amounts of fried catfish may increase the risk of weight gain and other health problems due to its high calorie, fat, and salt content.

It is generally recommended for pregnant women to consume fried catfish in moderation and to speak with their healthcare provider if they are concerned about the potential risks of consuming fried catfish. Pregnant women should also be aware of any food allergies or sensitivities they may have and should speak with their healthcare provider if they are concerned about the potential risks of consuming fried catfish.

Overall, fried catfish can be a tasty and convenient part of a healthy diet during pregnancy when consumed in moderation and with appropriate precautions. Pregnant women should speak with their healthcare provider about their dietary needs and any potential risks or concerns.

Fried chicken

Fried chicken is a type of chicken that is often prepared by coating thin slices of chicken in a mixture of flour, spices, and breadcrumbs, and then frying them in oil. Fried chicken is a popular food item that is often served as a snack or as part of a meal and is often enjoyed at restaurants, fast food chains, and other food establishments.

During pregnancy, it is generally considered safe to consume fried chicken in moderation as part of a healthy diet. However, it is important for pregnant women to be aware of the potential risks of consuming fried chicken, as well as the potential benefits.

Some pregnant women may be allergic to chicken or may have sensitivities to it. In addition, consuming large amounts of fried chicken may increase the risk of weight gain and other health problems due to its high calorie, fat, and salt content. Fried chicken is also often fried in oil, which can contribute to an unhealthy diet if consumed in large amounts.

It is generally recommended for pregnant women to consume fried chicken in moderation and to speak with their healthcare provider if they are concerned about the potential risks of consuming fried chicken. Pregnant women should also be aware of any food allergies or sensitivities they may have and should speak with their healthcare provider if they are concerned about the potential risks of consuming fried chicken.

Overall, fried chicken can be a tasty and convenient part of a healthy diet during pregnancy when consumed in moderation and with appropriate precautions. Pregnant women should speak with their healthcare provider about their dietary needs and any potential risks or concerns.

Fried rice

Fried rice is a popular dish that consists of cooked rice that is stir-fried with vegetables, meats, and other ingredients. Fried rice is often seasoned with soy sauce, sesame oil, and other spices and is typically served as a side dish or as a main meal.

During pregnancy, it is generally considered safe to consume fried rice as part of a healthy diet in moderation. Fried rice can be a good source of protein, carbohydrates, and other nutrients, and may have potential health benefits when consumed as part of a balanced diet.

However, it is important for pregnant women to be aware of the potential risks of consuming fried rice, as well as the potential benefits. Some pregnant women may be allergic to certain ingredients in fried rice or may have sensitivities to them. In addition, consuming large amounts of fried rice may increase the risk of weight gain and other health problems due to its high calorie and fat content.

It is generally recommended for pregnant women to consume fried rice in moderation and to speak with their healthcare provider if they are concerned about the potential risks of consuming fried rice. Pregnant women should also be aware of any food allergies or sensitivities they may have and should speak with their healthcare provider if they are concerned about the potential risks of consuming fried rice.

Overall, fried rice can be a tasty and convenient part of a healthy diet during pregnancy when consumed in moderation and with appropriate precautions. Pregnant women should speak with their healthcare provider about their dietary needs and any potential risks or concerns.

Frozen pizza

Frozen pizza is a type of pizza that is pre-made and then frozen for storage and transportation. Frozen pizzas are often sold in supermarkets and can be cooked at home in an oven or microwave. Frozen pizzas are a popular convenience food and are often seen as an easy and quick meal option.

During pregnancy, it is generally considered safe to consume frozen pizza in moderation as part of a healthy diet. Frozen pizza can be a good source of protein, carbohydrates, and other nutrients, and may have potential health benefits when consumed as part of a balanced diet.

However, it is important for pregnant women to be aware of the potential risks of consuming frozen pizza, as well as the potential benefits. Some frozen pizzas may contain ingredients that are not recommended for pregnant women, such as processed meats or high levels of sodium. In addition, consuming large amounts of frozen pizza may increase the risk of weight gain and other health problems due to its high calorie and fat content.

It is generally recommended for pregnant women to consume frozen pizza in moderation and to speak with their healthcare provider if they are concerned about the potential risks of consuming frozen pizza. Pregnant women should also be aware of any food allergies or sensitivities they may have and should speak with their healthcare provider if they are concerned about the potential risks of consuming frozen pizza.

Overall, frozen pizza can be a tasty and convenient part of a healthy diet during pregnancy when consumed in moderation and with appropriate precautions. Pregnant women should speak with their healthcare provider about their dietary needs and any potential risks or concerns.

Frozen waffles

Frozen waffles are a type of breakfast food that are made from a mixture of flour, eggs, milk, and other ingredients, and are cooked in a waffle iron. Frozen waffles are often sold in supermarkets and can be cooked at home in a toaster or oven. Frozen waffles are a popular convenience food and are often seen as an easy and quick breakfast option.

During pregnancy, it is generally considered safe to consume frozen waffles in moderation as part of a healthy diet. Frozen waffles can be a good source of protein, carbohydrates, and other nutrients, and may have potential health benefits when consumed as part of a balanced diet.

However, it is important for pregnant women to be aware of the potential risks of consuming frozen waffles, as well as the potential benefits. Some frozen waffles may contain ingredients that are not recommended for pregnant women, such as high levels of sodium or added sugars. In addition, consuming large amounts of frozen waffles may increase the risk of weight gain and other health problems due to their high calorie and fat content.

It is generally recommended for pregnant women to consume frozen waffles in moderation and to speak with their healthcare provider if they are concerned about the potential risks of consuming frozen waffles. Pregnant women should also be aware of any food allergies or sensitivities they may have and should speak with their healthcare provider if they are concerned about the potential risks of consuming frozen waffles.

Overall, frozen waffles can be a tasty and convenient part of a healthy diet during pregnancy when consumed in moderation and with appropriate precautions. Pregnant women should speak with their healthcare provider about their dietary needs and any potential risks or concerns.

Fruits and vegetables

It is generally recommended that pregnant women wash all fruits and vegetables before consuming them. This is because unwashed fruits and vegetables can contain harmful bacteria and other contaminants that can cause foodborne illness.

Pregnant women are at increased risk of foodborne illness because their immune systems are compromised during pregnancy. Consuming contaminated fruits and vegetables can increase the risk of contracting a bacterial infection, such as salmonella or E. coli. These infections can cause serious complications, including miscarriage, stillbirth, and severe illness in the mother.

To reduce the risk of foodborne illness, it is important for pregnant women to follow safe food handling practices, including washing their hands thoroughly with soap and water before handling food and washing all fruits and vegetables thoroughly before consuming them. Pregnant women should also be cautious about consuming other types of raw or undercooked products, such as raw sprouts, uncooked or undercooked meats, poultry, seafood, and eggs, and unpasteurized milk and dairy products.

In summary, it is generally recommended that pregnant women wash all fruits and vegetables before consuming them to reduce the risk of contracting a bacterial infection. Pregnant women should also follow safe food handling practices and be cautious about consuming other types of raw or undercooked products.

Garlic

Garlic is a type of herb that is widely used in cooking and is known for its pungent flavor and potential health benefits. Garlic is a good source of antioxidants and has been shown to have anti-inflammatory and immune-boosting properties.

During pregnancy, it is generally considered safe to consume garlic as part of a healthy diet. Garlic is a good source of nutrients that are important for the health and well-being of pregnant women, and may have potential benefits for certain health conditions, such as high blood pressure and cholesterol.

However, it is important for pregnant women to be aware of the potential risks of consuming garlic, as well as the potential benefits. Some pregnant women may be allergic to garlic or may have sensitivities to it. In addition, consuming large amounts of garlic may cause heartburn or other digestive problems in some individuals.

It is generally recommended for pregnant women to consume garlic in moderation and to speak with their healthcare provider if they are concerned about the potential risks of consuming garlic. Pregnant women should also be aware of any food allergies or sensitivities they may have and should speak with their healthcare provider if they are concerned about the potential risks of consuming garlic.

Overall, garlic can be a nutritious and flavorful part of a healthy diet during pregnancy when consumed in moderation and with appropriate precautions. Pregnant women should speak with their healthcare provider about their dietary needs and any potential risks or concerns.

Garlic bread

Garlic bread is a type of bread that is topped with a mixture of garlic, butter, and other ingredients, and is then baked or grilled until toasted. Garlic bread is often served as a side dish or as an accompaniment to main meals.

During pregnancy, it is generally considered safe to consume garlic bread in moderation as part of a healthy diet. Garlic bread can be a good source of carbohydrates and other nutrients, and may have potential health benefits when consumed as part of a balanced diet. Garlic, in particular, is a source of antioxidants and has been associated with a number of potential health benefits, including reducing the risk of heart disease and cancer.

However, it is important for pregnant women to be aware of the potential risks of consuming garlic bread, as well as the potential benefits. Some pregnant women may be allergic to garlic or may have sensitivities to it. In addition, consuming large amounts of garlic bread may increase the risk of weight gain and other health problems due to its high calorie and fat content.

It is generally recommended for pregnant women to consume garlic bread in moderation and to speak with their healthcare provider if they are concerned about the potential risks of consuming garlic bread. Pregnant women should also be aware of any food allergies or sensitivities they may have and should speak with their healthcare provider if they are concerned about the potential risks of consuming garlic bread.

Overall, garlic bread can be a tasty and convenient part of a healthy diet during pregnancy when consumed in moderation and with appropriate precautions. Pregnant women should speak with their healthcare provider about their dietary needs and any potential risks or concerns.

Ghee

Ghee is a type of clarified butter that is popular in Indian and other South Asian cuisines. It is made by simmering butter until the water and milk solids separate from the fat, and then straining out the solids. Ghee has a high smoke point and is often used for frying and cooking at high temperatures.

During pregnancy, it is generally considered safe to consume ghee in moderation as part of a healthy diet. Ghee is a source of fat and can be a good source of energy for pregnant women. Some studies have also suggested that ghee may have potential health benefits when consumed in moderation, including improving digestion and reducing the risk of heart disease.

However, it is important for pregnant women to be aware of the potential risks of consuming ghee, as well as the potential benefits. Ghee is high in fat and calories, and consuming large amounts of ghee may increase the risk of weight gain and other health problems. In addition, ghee may contain trace amounts of lactose, which may be problematic for pregnant women who are lactose intolerant.

It is generally recommended for pregnant women to consume ghee in moderation and to speak with their healthcare provider if they are concerned about the potential risks of consuming ghee.

Pregnant women should also be aware of any food allergies or sensitivities they may have and should speak with their healthcare provider if they are concerned about the potential risks of consuming ghee.

Overall, ghee can be a tasty and convenient part of a healthy diet during pregnancy when consumed in moderation and with appropriate precautions. Pregnant women should speak with their healthcare provider about their dietary needs and any potential risks or concerns.

Ginger for nausea

Ginger is a type of herb that is commonly used in cooking and has been used for centuries for its potential health benefits, including its ability to alleviate nausea and vomiting. Ginger is available in a variety of forms, including fresh, dried, and in supplement form, and can be consumed in a variety of ways, including as a spice in cooking, as a tea, or in capsule form.

During pregnancy, it is generally considered safe to consume ginger in small amounts as a natural remedy for nausea and vomiting. Some research suggests that ginger may be effective in reducing nausea and vomiting during pregnancy, particularly in the early stages.

However, it is important for pregnant women to be aware of the potential risks of consuming ginger, as well as the potential benefits. Some pregnant women may be allergic to ginger or may have sensitivities to it. In addition, consuming large amounts of ginger may cause heartburn or other digestive problems in some individuals.

It is generally recommended for pregnant women to consume ginger in moderation and to speak with their healthcare provider before using ginger as a natural remedy for nausea and vomiting. Pregnant women should also be aware of any food allergies or sensitivities they may have and should speak with their healthcare provider if they are concerned about the potential risks of consuming ginger.

Overall, ginger can be a useful natural remedy for nausea and vomiting during pregnancy when consumed in small amounts and with appropriate medical supervision. Pregnant women should speak with their healthcare provider about the appropriate use of ginger as a natural remedy for nausea and vomiting and about any potential risks or concerns.

Grapes

Grapes are a type of fruit that are native to the Mediterranean region and are widely cultivated around the world. Grapes are a good source of nutrients, including vitamins, minerals, and antioxidants, and are available in a variety of forms, including fresh, frozen, dried, and as juice.

During pregnancy, it is generally considered safe to consume grapes as part of a healthy diet. Grapes are a good source of nutrients that are important for the health and well-being of pregnant women, including vitamins C and K, potassium, and fiber. Grapes may also have potential benefits for certain health conditions, such as high blood pressure and constipation.

However, it is important for pregnant women to be aware of the potential risks of consuming grapes, as well as the potential benefits. Some pregnant women may be allergic to grapes or may have sensitivities to them. In addition, consuming large amounts of grapes may cause heartburn or other digestive problems in some individuals.

It is generally recommended for pregnant women to consume grapes in moderation and to speak with their healthcare provider if they are concerned about the potential risks of consuming grapes. Pregnant women should also be aware of any food allergies or sensitivities they may have and should speak with their healthcare provider if they are concerned about the potential risks of consuming grapes.

Overall, grapes can be a nutritious and flavorful part of a healthy diet during pregnancy when consumed in moderation and with appropriate precautions. Pregnant women should speak with their healthcare provider about their dietary needs and any potential risks or concerns.

Green beans

Green beans, also known as string beans or snap beans, are a type of legume that is widely cultivated and consumed around the world. Green beans are a good source of nutrients, including vitamins, minerals, and fiber, and are available in a variety of forms, including fresh, frozen, and canned.

During pregnancy, it is generally considered safe to consume green beans as part of a healthy diet. Green beans are a good source of nutrients that are important for the health and well-being of pregnant women, including vitamins A, C, and K, potassium, and fiber. Green beans may also have potential benefits for certain health conditions, such as constipation and high blood pressure.

However, it is important for pregnant women to be aware of the potential risks of consuming green beans, as well as the potential benefits. Some pregnant women may be allergic to green beans or may have sensitivities to them. In addition, consuming large amounts of green beans may cause heartburn or other digestive problems in some individuals.

It is generally recommended for pregnant women to consume green beans in moderation and to speak with their healthcare provider if they are concerned about the potential risks of consuming green beans. Pregnant women should also be aware of any food allergies or sensitivities they may have and should speak with their healthcare provider if they are concerned about the potential risks of consuming green beans.

Overall, green beans can be a nutritious and flavorful part of a healthy diet during pregnancy when consumed in moderation and with appropriate precautions. Pregnant women should speak with their healthcare provider about their dietary needs and any potential risks or concerns.

Grits

Grits are a type of cornmeal that is ground into a coarse, granular texture and cooked with water or milk to create a porridge-like dish. Grits are a staple food in the southern United States and are often served as a breakfast food, but they can also be used as a base for savory dishes or as a side dish.

During pregnancy, it is generally considered safe to consume grits as part of a healthy diet. Grits are a good source of carbohydrates and can provide energy for pregnant women. They are also a source of several nutrients, including iron, folate, and B vitamins.

However, it is important for pregnant women to be aware of the potential risks of consuming grits, as well as the potential benefits. Some grits may be enriched with added nutrients, such as folic acid, which is important for fetal development. However, some grits may also contain added sugars or sodium, which may not be recommended for pregnant women in large amounts. In addition, consuming large amounts of grits may increase the risk of weight gain and other health problems due to their high calorie and fat content.

It is generally recommended for pregnant women to consume grits in moderation and to speak with their healthcare provider if they are concerned about the potential risks of consuming grits. Pregnant women should also be aware of any food allergies or sensitivities they may have and should speak with their healthcare provider if they are concerned about the potential risks of consuming grits.

Overall, grits can be a tasty and convenient part of a healthy diet during pregnancy when consumed in moderation and with appropriate precautions. Pregnant women should speak with their healthcare provider about their dietary needs and any potential risks or concerns.

Guacamole

Guacamole is a popular Mexican dip or spread made from mashed avocados, diced onions, diced tomatoes, lime juice, and various herbs and spices. It is often served with tortilla chips or used as a topping for tacos, burritos, and other Mexican dishes.

During pregnancy, it is generally considered safe to consume guacamole as part of a healthy diet. Avocados are a good source of healthy fats, fiber, and various nutrients, including potassium, folate, and vitamin K. These nutrients can be important for pregnant women, as they may help to support fetal development and overall health.

However, it is important for pregnant women to be aware of the potential risks of consuming guacamole, as well as the potential benefits. Some guacamole recipes may contain raw onions or raw garlic, which can increase the risk of food poisoning or other health problems if they are not handled or prepared properly. In addition, guacamole may contain added sugars, sodium, or other ingredients that may not be recommended for pregnant women in large amounts.

It is generally recommended for pregnant women to consume guacamole in moderation and to speak with their healthcare provider if they are concerned about the potential risks of consuming guacamole. Pregnant women should also be aware of any food allergies or sensitivities they may have and should speak with their healthcare provider if they are concerned about the potential risks of consuming guacamole.

Overall, guacamole can be a tasty and convenient part of a healthy diet during pregnancy when consumed in moderation and with appropriate precautions. Pregnant women should speak with

their healthcare provider about their dietary needs and any potential risks or concerns.

Hamburgers

A hamburger is a sandwich consisting of a patty of ground beef, usually cooked, placed inside a sliced bun or roll. Hamburger patties may be grilled, fried, or cooked in other ways, and they are often served with a variety of toppings such as lettuce, tomato, onions, pickles, cheese, ketchup, mustard, and mayonnaise.

During pregnancy, it is generally considered safe to consume hamburgers as part of a healthy diet, as long as they are cooked to a safe temperature and handled properly to reduce the risk of food poisoning or other health problems. Beef is a good source of protein, iron, and other nutrients, which can be important for pregnant women.

However, it is important for pregnant women to be aware of the potential risks of consuming hamburgers, as well as the potential benefits. Some hamburgers may be high in saturated fat, sodium, or added sugars, which may not be recommended for pregnant women in large amounts. In addition, consuming large amounts of hamburgers or other processed meats may increase the risk of certain health problems, such as heart disease or cancer.

It is generally recommended for pregnant women to consume hamburgers in moderation and to speak with their healthcare provider if they are concerned about the potential risks of consuming hamburgers. Pregnant women should also be aware of any food allergies or sensitivities they may have and should speak with their healthcare provider if they are concerned about the potential risks of consuming hamburgers.

Overall, hamburgers can be a tasty and convenient part of a healthy diet during pregnancy when consumed in moderation and with appropriate precautions. Pregnant women should speak with

their healthcare provider about their dietary needs and any potential risks or concerns.

Ham

Ham is a type of cured and cooked pork that is often consumed as a meat in sandwiches, as a topping for pizzas, or as a main dish. There are many different types of ham available, including country ham, city ham, and honey-baked ham, which vary in flavor and preparation methods.

During pregnancy, it is generally considered safe to consume ham as part of a healthy diet, as long as it is cooked to a safe temperature and handled properly to reduce the risk of food poisoning or other health problems. Pork is a good source of protein, iron, and other nutrients, which can be important for pregnant women.

However, it is important for pregnant women to be aware of the potential risks of consuming ham, as well as the potential benefits. Some types of ham may be high in sodium, added sugars, or other ingredients that may not be recommended for pregnant women in large amounts. In addition, consuming large amounts of ham or other processed meats may increase the risk of certain health problems, such as heart disease or cancer.

It is generally recommended for pregnant women to consume ham in moderation and to speak with their healthcare provider if they are concerned about the potential risks of consuming ham. Pregnant women should also be aware of any food allergies or sensitivities they may have and should speak with their healthcare provider if they are concerned about the potential risks of consuming ham.

Overall, ham can be a tasty and convenient part of a healthy diet during pregnancy when consumed in moderation and with appropriate precautions. Pregnant women should speak with their healthcare provider about their dietary needs and any potential risks or concerns.

Hot dogs

Hot dogs are a type of processed meat, usually made from beef, pork, chicken, or a combination of these meats, that is formed into a sausage shape and cooked. Hot dogs are often served in a bun or roll and may be topped with a variety of condiments such as ketchup, mustard, onions, relish, cheese, and mayonnaise.

During pregnancy, it is generally considered safe to consume hot dogs as part of a healthy diet, as long as they are cooked to a safe temperature and handled properly to reduce the risk of food poisoning or other health problems. Processed meats like hot dogs are good sources of protein, iron, and other nutrients, which can be important for pregnant women.

However, it is important for pregnant women to be aware of the potential risks of consuming hot dogs, as well as the potential benefits. Some hot dogs may be high in sodium, added sugars, or other ingredients that may not be recommended for pregnant women in large amounts. In addition, consuming large amounts of hot dogs or other processed meats may increase the risk of certain health problems, such as heart disease or cancer.

It is generally recommended for pregnant women to consume hot dogs in moderation and to speak with their healthcare provider if they are concerned about the potential risks of consuming hot dogs. Pregnant women should also be aware of any food allergies or sensitivities they may have and should speak with their healthcare provider if they are concerned about the potential risks of consuming hot dogs.

Overall, hot dogs can be a tasty and convenient part of a healthy diet during pregnancy when consumed in moderation and with appropriate precautions. Pregnant women should speak with their healthcare provider about their dietary needs and any potential risks or concerns.

Hummus

Hummus is a Middle Eastern dip or spread made from mashed chickpeas, tahini (a paste made from sesame seeds), lemon juice, and garlic. Hummus is often seasoned with spices such as cumin and paprika and may be served with vegetables, bread, or crackers as a snack or appetizer.

During pregnancy, hummus can be a healthy and nutritious food to include in a well-balanced diet. Chickpeas, the main ingredient in hummus, are a good source of protein, fiber, and other nutrients, including iron, folate, and zinc, which can be important for pregnant women. In addition, hummus is often made with tahini, which is a good source of calcium and other nutrients, and lemon juice, which is a good source of vitamin C.

However, it is important for pregnant women to be aware of the potential risks of consuming hummus, as well as the potential benefits. Some hummus products may be high in sodium or other ingredients that may not be recommended for pregnant women in large amounts. In addition, pregnant women should be aware of any food allergies or sensitivities they may have and should speak with their healthcare provider if they are concerned about the potential risks of consuming hummus.

Overall, hummus can be a tasty and nutritious part of a healthy diet during pregnancy when consumed in moderation and with appropriate precautions. Pregnant women should speak with their healthcare provider about their dietary needs and any potential risks or concerns.

Ice cream

Ice cream is a frozen dessert made from a mixture of cream, milk, sugar, and flavorings, such as fruit, nuts, chocolate, or caramel. Ice cream may also contain other ingredients, such as stabilizers, emulsifiers, and preservatives, to improve its texture and flavor.

During pregnancy, ice cream can be enjoyed as part of a healthy and balanced diet, as long as it is consumed in moderation and as part of an overall healthy eating pattern. Ice cream is a good source of calcium and other nutrients, which can be important for pregnant women. However, ice cream is also high in fat, sugar, and calories, and consuming large amounts of ice cream or other high-fat, high-sugar foods may contribute to weight gain and other health problems during pregnancy.

It is generally recommended for pregnant women to consume ice cream in moderation and to choose low-fat or reduced-sugar options when possible. Pregnant women should also be aware of any food allergies or sensitivities they may have and should speak with their healthcare provider if they are concerned about the potential risks of consuming ice cream.

Overall, ice cream can be a tasty and enjoyable part of a healthy diet during pregnancy when consumed in moderation and with appropriate precautions. Pregnant women should speak with their healthcare provider about their dietary needs and any potential risks or concerns.

Ice cream sandwiches

Ice cream sandwiches are a frozen dessert made from two thin, flat cookies or wafers sandwiching a layer of ice cream. Ice cream sandwiches may also contain other ingredients, such as chocolate, caramel, or nuts, to improve their flavor and texture.

During pregnancy, ice cream sandwiches can be enjoyed as part of a healthy and balanced diet, as long as they are consumed in moderation and as part of an overall healthy eating pattern. Ice cream sandwiches may be a good source of calcium and other nutrients, which can be important for pregnant women. However, ice cream sandwiches are also high in fat, sugar, and calories, and consuming large amounts of ice cream sandwiches or other high-fat, high-sugar foods may contribute to weight gain and other health problems during pregnancy.

It is generally recommended for pregnant women to consume ice cream sandwiches in moderation and to choose low-fat or reduced-sugar options when possible. Pregnant women should also be aware of any food allergies or sensitivities they may have and should speak with their healthcare provider if they are concerned about the potential risks of consuming ice cream sandwiches.

Overall, ice cream sandwiches can be a tasty and enjoyable part of a healthy diet during pregnancy when consumed in moderation and with appropriate precautions. Pregnant women should speak with their healthcare provider about their dietary needs and any potential risks or concerns.

Jams and jellies

Jams and jellies are spreads made from fruit and sugar that are cooked together until thickened and then cooled and set. Jams and jellies may contain additional ingredients, such as pectin, a natural thickening agent found in fruits, or other preservatives, to improve their texture and stability.

During pregnancy, jams and jellies can be consumed as part of a healthy and balanced diet, as long as they are consumed in moderation and as part of an overall healthy eating pattern. Jams and jellies are a good source of vitamins, minerals, and antioxidants, which can be important for pregnant women. However, jams and jellies are also high in sugar, and consuming large amounts of jams and jellies or other high-sugar foods may contribute to weight gain and other health problems during pregnancy.

It is generally recommended for pregnant women to consume jams and jellies in moderation and to choose low-sugar or reduced-calorie options when possible. Pregnant women should also be aware of any food allergies or sensitivities they may have and should speak with their healthcare provider if they are concerned about the potential risks of consuming jams and jellies.

Overall, jams and jellies can be a tasty and enjoyable part of a healthy diet during pregnancy when consumed in moderation and with appropriate precautions. Pregnant women should speak with their healthcare provider about their dietary needs and any potential risks or concerns.

Jambalaya

Jambalaya is a traditional Creole dish from Louisiana, USA, made from a mixture of meats, vegetables, and rice that is seasoned with a variety of herbs and spices. Jambalaya is typically made with a combination of meats such as sausage, ham, chicken, or seafood, and vegetables such as onions, bell peppers, and celery. The ingredients are usually cooked together in a large pot or Dutch oven, and the dish is finished by adding cooked rice to the mixture.

During pregnancy, jambalaya can be consumed as part of a healthy and balanced diet, as long as it is prepared using safe food handling practices and cooked to a safe temperature. Jambalaya can be a good source of protein, vitamins, minerals, and other nutrients, which can be important for pregnant women. However, jambalaya may also contain ingredients that should be limited or avoided during pregnancy, such as high-fat meats, processed meats, and large amounts of salt.

It is generally recommended for pregnant women to choose lean proteins, such as chicken, turkey, or tofu, and to limit their intake of high-fat meats and processed meats during pregnancy. Pregnant women should also be mindful of their intake of salt and should choose low-sodium or reduced-salt options when possible. Pregnant women should also be aware of any food allergies or sensitivities they may have and should speak with their healthcare provider if they are concerned about the potential risks of consuming jambalaya.

Overall, jambalaya can be a tasty and enjoyable part of a healthy diet during pregnancy when consumed in moderation and with appropriate precautions. Pregnant women should speak with their healthcare provider about their dietary needs and any potential risks or concerns.

Kale

Kale is a type of leafy green vegetable that belongs to the cabbage family and is native to the eastern Mediterranean and Asia Minor. Kale is a good source of nutrients, including vitamins, minerals, and antioxidants, and is available in a variety of forms, including fresh, frozen, and canned.

During pregnancy, it is generally considered safe to consume kale as part of a healthy diet. Kale is a good source of nutrients that are important for the health and well-being of pregnant women, including vitamins K, A, and C, potassium, and calcium. Kale may also have potential benefits for certain health conditions, such as constipation, high blood pressure, and anemia.

However, it is important for pregnant women to be aware of the potential risks of consuming kale, as well as the potential benefits. Some pregnant women may be allergic to kale or may have sensitivities to it. In addition, consuming large amounts of kale may cause heartburn or other digestive problems in some individuals.

It is generally recommended for pregnant women to consume kale in moderation and to speak with their healthcare provider if they are concerned about the potential risks of consuming kale. Pregnant women should also be aware of any food allergies or sensitivities they may have and should speak with their healthcare provider if they are concerned about the potential risks of consuming kale.

Overall, kale can be a nutritious and flavorful part of a healthy diet during pregnancy when consumed in moderation and with appropriate precautions. Pregnant women should speak with their healthcare provider about their dietary needs and any potential risks or concerns.

Ketchup

Ketchup is a condiment made from tomatoes, vinegar, sugar, and a variety of spices and flavorings. It is commonly used to add flavor and moisture to a variety of dishes, including burgers, hot dogs, sandwiches, and fries.

During pregnancy, ketchup can be consumed as part of a healthy and balanced diet, as long as it is consumed in moderation and as part of an overall healthy eating pattern. Ketchup is a good source of vitamins, minerals, and antioxidants, which can be important for pregnant women. However, ketchup is also high in sugar and sodium, and consuming large amounts of ketchup or other high-sugar or high-sodium foods may contribute to weight gain and other health problems during pregnancy.

It is generally recommended for pregnant women to consume ketchup in moderation and to choose low-sugar or low-sodium options when possible. Pregnant women should also be mindful of their intake of added sugars and sodium and should aim to limit their intake of these nutrients during pregnancy. Pregnant women should also be aware of any food allergies or sensitivities they may have and should speak with their healthcare provider if they are concerned about the potential risks of consuming ketchup.

Overall, ketchup can be a tasty and enjoyable part of a healthy diet during pregnancy when consumed in moderation and with appropriate precautions. Pregnant women should speak with their healthcare provider about their dietary needs and any potential risks or concerns.

Leeks

Leeks are a type of vegetable that belong to the onion family and are native to the eastern Mediterranean and Asia Minor. Leeks are a good source of nutrients, including vitamins, minerals, and antioxidants, and are available in a variety of forms, including fresh, frozen, and canned.

During pregnancy, it is generally considered safe to consume leeks as part of a healthy diet. Leeks are a good source of nutrients that are important for the health and well-being of pregnant women, including vitamins K and C, folate, and potassium. Leeks may also have potential benefits for certain health conditions, such as high blood pressure, anemia, and constipation.

However, it is important for pregnant women to be aware of the potential risks of consuming leeks, as well as the potential benefits. Some pregnant women may be allergic to leeks or may have sensitivities to them. In addition, consuming large amounts of leeks may cause heartburn or other digestive problems in some individuals.

It is generally recommended for pregnant women to consume leeks in moderation and to speak with their healthcare provider if they are concerned about the potential risks of consuming leeks. Pregnant women should also be aware of any food allergies or sensitivities they may have and should speak with their healthcare provider if they are concerned about the potential risks of consuming leeks.

Overall, leeks can be a nutritious and flavorful part of a healthy diet during pregnancy when consumed in moderation and with appropriate precautions. Pregnant women should speak with their healthcare provider about their dietary needs and any potential risks or concerns.

Leg of lamb

Leg of lamb is a cut of lamb meat taken from the hind leg of the animal. It is typically roasted or grilled and can be served as a main dish or used in a variety of dishes, such as stews, roasts, and sandwiches.

During pregnancy, leg of lamb can be consumed as part of a healthy and balanced diet, as long as it is prepared using safe food handling practices and cooked to a safe temperature. Lamb is a good source of protein, vitamins, minerals, and other nutrients, which can be important for pregnant women. However, lamb may also contain high levels of fat and cholesterol, and consuming large amounts of lamb or other high-fat meats may contribute to weight gain and other health problems during pregnancy.

It is generally recommended for pregnant women to choose lean proteins, such as chicken, turkey, or tofu, and to limit their intake of high-fat meats during pregnancy. Pregnant women should also be mindful of their intake of cholesterol and should choose cuts of lamb that are leaner and lower in fat and cholesterol when possible. Pregnant women should also be aware of any food allergies or sensitivities they may have and should speak with their healthcare provider if they are concerned about the potential risks of consuming leg of lamb.

Overall, leg of lamb can be a tasty and enjoyable part of a healthy diet during pregnancy when consumed in moderation and with appropriate precautions. Pregnant women should speak with their healthcare provider about their dietary needs and any potential risks or concerns.

Legumes

Legumes are a type of plant that belongs to the pea family and includes a wide variety of foods, such as beans, lentils, chickpeas, and peas. Legumes are a good source of nutrients, including proteins, fibers, and complex carbohydrates, and are available in a variety of forms, including fresh, frozen, and canned.

During pregnancy, it is generally considered safe to consume legumes as part of a healthy diet. Legumes are a good source of nutrients that are important for the health and well-being of pregnant women, including proteins, fibers, folate, and iron. Legumes may also have potential benefits for certain health conditions, such as constipation, high blood pressure, and anemia.

However, it is important for pregnant women to be aware of the potential risks of consuming legumes, as well as the potential benefits. Some pregnant women may be allergic to legumes or may have sensitivities to them. In addition, consuming large amounts of legumes may cause heartburn or other digestive problems in some individuals.

It is generally recommended for pregnant women to consume legumes in moderation and to speak with their healthcare provider if they are concerned about the potential risks of consuming legumes. Pregnant women should also be aware of any food allergies or sensitivities they may have and should speak with their healthcare provider if they are concerned about the potential risks of consuming legumes.

Overall, legumes can be a nutritious and flavorful part of a healthy diet during pregnancy when consumed in moderation and with appropriate precautions. Pregnant women should speak with their healthcare provider about their dietary needs and any potential risks or concerns.

Lemonade

Lemonade is a sweetened beverage made from lemon juice, water, and sugar. It can be served cold or hot and is often flavored with other ingredients, such as herbs, spices, or fruit juices.

During pregnancy, lemonade can be consumed as part of a healthy and balanced diet, as long as it is made with safe ingredients and consumed in moderation. Lemonade can be a good source of vitamin C, which is important for pregnant women, as it helps to support the immune system and promote healthy skin and tissues. However, lemonade may also contain high amounts of sugar, which can contribute to weight gain and other health problems during pregnancy.

It is generally recommended for pregnant women to limit their intake of sugary drinks, including lemonade, and to choose water and other unsweetened beverages instead. Pregnant women should also be mindful of their intake of added sugars and should choose lemonade that is made with minimal or no added sugars when possible. Pregnant women should also be aware of any food allergies or sensitivities they may have and should speak with their healthcare provider if they are concerned about the potential risks of consuming lemonade.

Overall, lemonade can be a tasty and refreshing beverage during pregnancy when consumed in moderation and with appropriate precautions. Pregnant women should speak with their healthcare provider about their dietary needs and any potential risks or concerns.

Lentils

Lentils are a type of legume that belongs to the pea family and is native to the eastern Mediterranean and Asia Minor. Lentils are a good source of nutrients, including proteins, fibers, and complex carbohydrates, and are available in a variety of forms, including fresh, frozen, and canned.

During pregnancy, it is generally considered safe to consume lentils as part of a healthy diet. Lentils are a good source of nutrients that are important for the health and well-being of pregnant women, including proteins, fibers, folate, and iron. Lentils may also have potential benefits for certain health conditions, such as constipation, high blood pressure, and anemia.

However, it is important for pregnant women to be aware of the potential risks of consuming lentils, as well as the potential benefits. Some pregnant women may be allergic to lentils or may have sensitivities to them. In addition, consuming large amounts of lentils may cause heartburn or other digestive problems in some individuals.

It is generally recommended for pregnant women to consume lentils in moderation and to speak with their healthcare provider if they are concerned about the potential risks of consuming lentils. Pregnant women should also be aware of any food allergies or sensitivities they may have and should speak with their healthcare provider if they are concerned about the potential risks of consuming lentils.

Overall, lentils can be a nutritious and flavorful part of a healthy diet during pregnancy when consumed in moderation and with appropriate precautions. Pregnant women should speak with their healthcare provider about their dietary needs and any potential risks or concerns.

Licorice

Licorice is a sweet and flavorful herb that is commonly used to make candy and other sweet treats. It is made from the root of the Glycyrrhiza glabra plant and has a characteristic black or dark brown color and a sweet, slightly bitter flavor. Licorice is often used in folk medicine as a natural remedy for various health problems, including indigestion, sore throat, and cough.

During pregnancy, licorice can be consumed in small amounts as part of a healthy and balanced diet. However, it is important to be aware that licorice can have some potential risks and side effects when consumed in large amounts or over long periods of time.

One of the main concerns with licorice during pregnancy is that it may contain high levels of glycyrrhizin, a compound that can increase blood pressure and cause fluid retention in some people. High blood pressure and fluid retention can be harmful for pregnant women, as they may increase the risk of complications such as preterm labor and low birth weight.

In addition, some studies have suggested that licorice may interfere with the absorption and metabolism of certain medications, including drugs used to treat high blood pressure, diabetes, and heart disease. Pregnant women who are taking medications or have underlying health conditions should be particularly cautious about consuming licorice and should speak with their healthcare provider about the potential risks and benefits.

Overall, licorice can be a tasty and enjoyable treat during pregnancy when consumed in moderation and with appropriate precautions. Pregnant women should be mindful of their intake of licorice and should speak with their healthcare provider if they are concerned about the potential risks.

Lima beans

Lima beans, also known as butter beans, are a type of legume that is generally considered safe to eat during pregnancy. Like other legumes, lima beans are a good source of protein, fiber, and various nutrients, including folate, iron, and zinc, which are important for fetal development and the health of the mother.

However, it is important to follow proper food safety guidelines when consuming lima beans or any other legumes during pregnancy. This includes cooking the beans thoroughly to reduce the risk of foodborne illness, and discarding any beans that are spoiled or show signs of spoilage.

In addition, it is recommended to avoid consuming large amounts of lima beans or other legumes if you have a history of kidney stones, as these foods are high in oxalates and may increase the risk of developing kidney stones.

Overall, lima beans can be a healthy and nutritious addition to the diet of a pregnant woman, as long as they are properly prepared and consumed in moderation.

Liver and other vitamin A-rich foods

Vitamin A is an important nutrient that is essential for fetal development and the health of the mother during pregnancy. However, it is important to consume vitamin A in the right amounts during pregnancy, as too much vitamin A can be harmful to the developing fetus.

Liver is a rich source of vitamin A, and it is generally considered safe to eat small amounts of liver during pregnancy. However, it is not recommended to consume large amounts of liver or other vitamin A-rich foods, such as cod liver oil, during pregnancy, as this can lead to an excess intake of vitamin A, which can be harmful to the developing fetus.

The recommended daily intake of vitamin A during pregnancy is 700-900 micrograms (mcg) per day. It is generally safe to consume up to 10,000 mcg of vitamin A per day from plant-based sources, such as fruits and vegetables, but it is not recommended to consume more than this amount.

To ensure an adequate intake of vitamin A during pregnancy, it is recommended to consume a varied and balanced diet that includes a variety of sources of vitamin A, such as sweet potatoes, carrots, spinach, and fortified foods, such as milk and cereals. It is also a good idea to consult with a healthcare provider or a registered dietitian for personalized nutrition advice.

Macaroni and cheese

Macaroni and cheese is a popular and comforting dish made from pasta and a creamy cheese sauce. It is often made with elbow macaroni, cheddar cheese, and milk, and can be served hot or cold. Macaroni and cheese can be a quick and easy meal or snack option and is often enjoyed by people of all ages.

During pregnancy, macaroni and cheese can be consumed as part of a healthy and balanced diet, as long as it is made with safe and nutritious ingredients and consumed in moderation. Macaroni and cheese can be a good source of protein, carbohydrates, and certain nutrients, such as calcium and vitamin D, which are important for pregnant women.

However, it is important to be mindful of the type and quality of ingredients used to make macaroni and cheese, as some versions may be high in fat, salt, and added sugars. Pregnant women should choose macaroni and cheese made with whole grain pasta, low-fat or fat-free milk, and reduced-fat cheese when possible. They should also be mindful of their intake of added sugars and should choose macaroni and cheese that is made with minimal or no added sugars when possible.

In addition, pregnant women should be aware of any food allergies or sensitivities they may have and should speak with their healthcare provider if they are concerned about the potential risks of consuming macaroni and cheese.

Overall, macaroni and cheese can be a tasty and satisfying meal or snack option during pregnancy when consumed in moderation and with appropriate precautions. Pregnant women should speak with their healthcare provider about their dietary needs and any potential risks or concerns.

Mangos

Mangos are generally considered safe to eat during pregnancy. They are a good source of several essential nutrients, including vitamin C, vitamin A, and potassium, which are important for fetal development and the health of the mother.

However, it is important to follow proper food safety guidelines when consuming mangoes or any other produce during pregnancy. This includes washing the mangoes thoroughly to remove any dirt or contaminants, and discarding any mangoes that are spoiled or show signs of spoilage.

In addition, it is recommended to avoid consuming large amounts of mangoes or other fruits if you are prone to developing gestational diabetes, as these foods are high in natural sugars and may increase the risk of developing this condition.

Overall, mangoes can be a healthy and nutritious addition to the diet of a pregnant woman, as long as they are properly prepared and consumed in moderation.

Mango lassi

Mango lassi is a refreshing and flavorful drink that is popular in South Asia and other parts of the world. It is made with mango, yogurt, milk, and ice, and is often blended together until smooth and creamy. Mango lassi can be served cold or at room temperature and is often enjoyed as a refreshing and hydrating beverage.

During pregnancy, mango lassi can be a nutritious and enjoyable drink option, as long as it is made with safe and high-quality ingredients. Mango lassi can be a good source of nutrients such as protein, calcium, and vitamin D, which are important for pregnant women. Mango is also a good source of vitamin C, which is important for immune function and skin health.

However, it is important to be mindful of the type and quality of ingredients used to make mango lassi, as some versions may be high in added sugars or other sweeteners. Pregnant women should choose mango lassi made with low-fat or fat-free yogurt and milk, and minimal or no added sugars when possible. They should also be mindful of their intake of added sugars and should choose mango lassi that is made with minimal or no added sugars when possible.

In addition, pregnant women should be aware of any food allergies or sensitivities they may have and should speak with their healthcare provider if they are concerned about the potential risks of consuming mango lassi.

Overall, mango lassi can be a nutritious and tasty drink option during pregnancy when consumed in moderation and with appropriate precautions. Pregnant women should speak with their healthcare provider about their dietary needs and any potential risks or concerns.

Mango smoothie

Mango smoothies are a popular and refreshing beverage made with mango, milk, yogurt, and ice. They are often blended together until smooth and creamy and can be served cold or at room temperature. Mango smoothies can be a nutritious and enjoyable drink option, as long as they are made with safe and high-quality ingredients.

During pregnancy, mango smoothies can be a good source of nutrients such as protein, calcium, and vitamin D, which are important for pregnant women. Mango is also a good source of vitamin C, which is important for immune function and skin health.

However, it is important to be mindful of the type and quality of ingredients used to make mango smoothies, as some versions may be high in added sugars or other sweeteners. Pregnant women should choose mango smoothies made with low-fat or fat-free milk and yogurt, and minimal or no added sugars when possible. They should also be mindful of their intake of added sugars and should choose mango smoothies that are made with minimal or no added sugars when possible.

In addition, pregnant women should be aware of any food allergies or sensitivities they may have and should speak with their healthcare provider if they are concerned about the potential risks of consuming mango smoothies.

Overall, mango smoothies can be a nutritious and tasty drink option during pregnancy when consumed in moderation and with appropriate precautions. Pregnant women should speak with their healthcare provider about their dietary needs and any potential risks or concerns.

Maple syrup

Maple syrup is a sweet, amber-colored syrup that is made from the sap of maple trees. It is commonly used as a topping for pancakes, waffles, and other baked goods, and is also used in cooking and baking as a sweetener.

During pregnancy, maple syrup can be consumed in moderation as part of a healthy and balanced diet. Like other types of sugars, maple syrup is a source of empty calories, meaning it provides energy without any other important nutrients. Therefore, it is important to be mindful of your intake of maple syrup and to choose it as an occasional treat rather than a daily staple.

Pregnant women should aim to limit their intake of added sugars, including maple syrup, as excessive consumption of added sugars can contribute to excess weight gain and other negative health outcomes. The American Heart Association recommends that women consume no more than 100 calories per day (about 6 teaspoons) of added sugars during pregnancy.

In addition, pregnant women should be aware of any food allergies or sensitivities they may have and should speak with their healthcare provider if they are concerned about the potential risks of consuming maple syrup.

Overall, maple syrup can be a tasty and enjoyable addition to a healthy and balanced diet during pregnancy when consumed in moderation. Pregnant women should speak with their healthcare provider about their dietary needs and any potential risks or concerns.

Marinara sauce

Marinara sauce is a tomato-based sauce that is commonly used in Italian cooking. It is made with a combination of tomatoes, onions, garlic, and herbs, and is often used to top pasta, pizzas, and other dishes.

During pregnancy, marinara sauce can be a nutritious and flavorful addition to a healthy and balanced diet. Tomatoes, which are the main ingredient in marinara sauce, are a good source of vitamins and minerals, including vitamin C, potassium, and lycopene. Lycopene is a powerful antioxidant that has been shown to have a number of potential health benefits, including a reduced risk of certain types of cancer.

However, it is important to be mindful of the ingredients and additives used in marinara sauce, as some types may be high in added sugars, salt, or other additives. Pregnant women should choose marinara sauce made with minimal or no added sugars and salt when possible and should be mindful of their intake of these nutrients.

In addition, pregnant women should be aware of any food allergies or sensitivities they may have and should speak with their healthcare provider if they are concerned about the potential risks of consuming marinara sauce.

Overall, marinara sauce can be a nutritious and tasty addition to a healthy and balanced diet during pregnancy when consumed in moderation and with appropriate precautions. Pregnant women should speak with their healthcare provider about their dietary needs and any potential risks or concerns.

Marshmallows

Marshmallows are a sweet, fluffy confection made from sugar, corn syrup, water, and gelatin. They are often consumed as a snack or used as an ingredient in desserts, such as s'mores or rice krispie treats.

During pregnancy, marshmallows can be consumed in moderation as part of a healthy and balanced diet. Like other types of sweets, marshmallows are a source of empty calories, meaning they provide energy without any other important nutrients. Therefore, it is important to be mindful of your intake of marshmallows and to choose them as an occasional treat rather than a daily staple.

Pregnant women should aim to limit their intake of added sugars, including those found in marshmallows, as excessive consumption of added sugars can contribute to excess weight gain and other negative health outcomes. The American Heart Association recommends that women consume no more than 100 calories per day (about 6 teaspoons) of added sugars during pregnancy.

In addition, pregnant women should be aware of any food allergies or sensitivities they may have and should speak with their healthcare provider if they are concerned about the potential risks of consuming marshmallows. Some types of marshmallows may contain ingredients such as peanuts or other allergens, which can be harmful for some individuals.

Overall, marshmallows can be a tasty and enjoyable addition to a healthy and balanced diet during pregnancy when consumed in moderation. Pregnant women should speak with their healthcare provider about their dietary needs and any potential risks or concerns.

Massage therapy

Massage therapy can be a relaxing and therapeutic treatment for pregnant women. It can help to reduce stress and tension, improve circulation, and alleviate muscle aches and pains that may occur during pregnancy.

However, it is important to take certain precautions when receiving massage therapy during pregnancy. It is generally recommended to avoid lying on your back for extended periods of time during massage therapy, as this position can cause decreased blood flow to the uterus and may not be comfortable for the pregnant woman.

In addition, it is important to inform the massage therapist about the pregnancy and any specific concerns or medical conditions that may affect the massage treatment. The therapist can then adjust the massage techniques and pressure to ensure the safety and comfort of the pregnant woman.

Overall, massage therapy can be a beneficial and enjoyable treatment for pregnant women, as long as it is performed by a trained and licensed therapist and appropriate precautions are taken. It is a good idea to consult with a healthcare provider or a trained and licensed massage therapist for personalized recommendations and advice.

Melons such as watermelon and honeydew

Melons, such as watermelon and honeydew, are generally considered safe to eat during pregnancy. They are good sources of several essential nutrients, including vitamin C, potassium, and folate, which are important for fetal development and the health of the mother.

However, it is important to follow proper food safety guidelines when consuming melons or any other produce during pregnancy. This includes washing the melons thoroughly to remove any dirt or contaminants, and discarding any melons that are spoiled or show signs of spoilage.

In addition, it is recommended to avoid consuming large amounts of melons or other fruits if you are prone to developing gestational diabetes, as these foods are high in natural sugars and may increase the risk of developing this condition.

Overall, melons can be a healthy and nutritious addition to the diet of a pregnant woman, as long as they are properly prepared and consumed in moderation.

Meringue

Meringue is a type of sweet, fluffy confection made from whipped egg whites and sugar. It is often used as a topping for desserts, such as pies and cakes, or baked on its own to create meringue cookies or other treats.

Pregnant women can safely consume meringue as part of a healthy and balanced diet. However, they should be mindful of the following factors when deciding whether to include meringue in their diet:

- Nutrient content: Meringue is generally a low-calorie, low-fat food that is relatively low in nutrients. However, it can be a good source of protein, as it is made from egg whites.

- Allergies and sensitivities: Pregnant women with food allergies or sensitivities should be careful when consuming meringue, as it may contain ingredients that they are sensitive to. For example, some meringue is made with wheat, which can cause allergic reactions in some people. Pregnant women should be sure to read ingredient labels carefully and speak with their healthcare provider if they have any concerns.

- Sugar content: Meringue is made with sugar, which can contribute to weight gain and other health problems during pregnancy if consumed in excess. Pregnant women should be mindful of their sugar intake and choose meringue treats that are lower in sugar or make their own meringue using a sugar substitute.

Overall, pregnant women can safely consume meringue as part of a healthy and balanced diet. However, they should be mindful of the potential risks and consider the factors outlined above when deciding whether to include meringue in their diet.

Muffins

Muffins are a type of baked goods made with flour, sugar, and eggs, and often flavored with fruit, nuts, or other ingredients. They are typically small, round, and sweet, and can be eaten as a breakfast food, snack, or dessert.

Pregnant women can safely consume muffins as part of a healthy and balanced diet. However, they should be mindful of the following factors when deciding whether to include muffins in their diet:

- Nutrient content: The nutrient content of muffins can vary widely depending on the ingredients used and the recipe. Some muffins may be relatively high in nutrients, such as whole grain muffins that are made with whole wheat flour and contain nuts, seeds, or other nutritious ingredients. Others may be lower in nutrients, such as muffins that are made with refined flour and are high in sugar. Pregnant women should choose muffins that are high in nutrients and low in added sugars.

- Allergies and sensitivities: Pregnant women with food allergies or sensitivities should be careful when consuming muffins, as they may contain ingredients that they are sensitive to. For example, some muffins are made with nuts, which can cause allergic reactions in some people. Pregnant women should be sure to read ingredient labels carefully and speak with their healthcare provider if they have any concerns.

- Sugar content: Muffins can be high in sugar, particularly if they are made with sweetened fruit or are topped with a sweet glaze or icing. Pregnant women should be mindful of their sugar intake and choose muffins that are lower in sugar or make their own muffins using a sugar substitute.

Overall, pregnant women can safely consume muffins as part of a healthy and balanced diet. However, they should be mindful of the potential risks and consider the factors outlined above when deciding whether to include muffins in their diet.

Milk

It is generally recommended that pregnant women be cautious about consuming unpasteurized milk and dairy products. This is because unpasteurized milk and dairy products can contain harmful bacteria and other contaminants that can cause foodborne illness.

Pregnant women are at increased risk of foodborne illness because their immune systems are compromised during pregnancy. Consuming contaminated unpasteurized milk and dairy products can increase the risk of contracting a bacterial infection, such as listeriosis or salmonella. These infections can cause serious complications, including miscarriage, stillbirth, and severe illness in the mother.

Pasteurization is a process that involves heating milk and dairy products to a high temperature to kill harmful bacteria. Pasteurized milk and dairy products are safe to consume because the pasteurization process removes the risk of bacterial contamination.

It is important for pregnant women to be aware of the risks of consuming unpasteurized products and to choose pasteurized options instead. Pregnant women should also be cautious about consuming other types of unpasteurized products, such as raw sprouts, raw eggs, and raw meat.

In summary, it is generally recommended that pregnant women be cautious about consuming unpasteurized milk and dairy products to reduce the risk of contracting a bacterial infection. Pregnant women should choose pasteurized milk and dairy products and be cautious about consuming other types of unpasteurized products.

Mustard

Mustard is a condiment made from the seeds of the mustard plant, which is a member of the cabbage family. It is typically made by grinding the seeds and mixing them with vinegar, salt, and other ingredients to create a paste or a dry powder. Mustard is commonly used as a condiment on sandwiches, hot dogs, and other foods, and it is also used as an ingredient in various dishes, such as sauces, marinades, and salad dressings.

Pregnant women can safely consume mustard as part of a healthy and balanced diet. However, they should be mindful of the following factors when deciding whether to include mustard in their diet:

- Nutrient content: Mustard is low in calories and fat, and it is a good source of some nutrients, such as selenium and magnesium. However, the nutrient content of mustard can vary depending on the ingredients used and the recipe. Some mustards may be high in sodium, and others may contain added sugars or other ingredients that are less healthy. Pregnant women should choose mustards that are low in sodium and added sugars and that are made with whole mustard seeds rather than mustard flour or other processed ingredients.

- Allergies and sensitivities: Pregnant women with food allergies or sensitivities should be careful when consuming mustard, as it may contain ingredients that they are sensitive to. For example, some mustards are made with nuts, which can cause allergic reactions in some people. Pregnant women should be sure to read ingredient labels carefully and speak with their healthcare provider if they have any concerns.

- Safety concerns: Mustard seeds and mustard plants are known to contain compounds that can cause allergic reactions in some people. In addition, some people may develop an intolerance to mustard or other condiments that contain mustard. Pregnant women who have a history of allergies or sensitivities should be cautious when consuming mustard and should speak with their healthcare provider if they have any concerns.

Overall, pregnant women can safely consume mustard as part of a healthy and balanced diet. However, they should be mindful of the potential risks and consider the factors outlined above when deciding whether to include mustard in their diet.

Mung beans

Mung beans are a type of legume that is generally considered safe to eat during pregnancy. Like other legumes, mung beans are a good source of protein, fiber, and various nutrients, including folate, iron, and zinc, which are important for fetal development and the health of the mother.

However, it is important to follow proper food safety guidelines when consuming mung beans or any other legumes during pregnancy. This includes cooking the beans thoroughly to reduce the risk of foodborne illness, and discarding any beans that are spoiled or show signs of spoilage.

In addition, it is recommended to avoid consuming large amounts of mung beans or other legumes if you have a history of kidney stones, as these foods are high in oxalates and may increase the risk of developing kidney stones.

Overall, mung beans can be a healthy and nutritious addition to the diet of a pregnant woman, as long as they are properly prepared and consumed in moderation.

Nectarines

Nectarines are generally considered safe to eat during pregnancy. They are a good source of several essential nutrients, including vitamin C, potassium, and fiber, which are important for fetal development and the health of the mother.

However, it is important to follow proper food safety guidelines when consuming nectarines or any other produce during pregnancy. This includes washing the nectarines thoroughly to remove any dirt or contaminants, and discarding any nectarines that are spoiled or show signs of spoilage.

In addition, it is recommended to avoid consuming large amounts of nectarines or other fruits if you are prone to developing gestational diabetes, as these foods are high in natural sugars and may increase the risk of developing this condition.

Overall, nectarines can be a healthy and nutritious addition to the diet of a pregnant woman, as long as they are properly prepared and consumed in moderation.

Nuts and seeds

Nuts and seeds are a nutritious and healthy part of a balanced diet for pregnant women. They are a good source of protein, fiber, and various nutrients, including essential fatty acids, vitamins, and minerals, which are important for fetal development and the health of the mother.

However, it is important to choose unsalted nuts and seeds during pregnancy to help control sodium intake and reduce the risk of high blood pressure. It is also a good idea to avoid consuming large amounts of nuts and seeds if you have a history of allergies, as these foods can trigger allergic reactions in some people.

In addition, it is recommended to avoid consuming large amounts of nuts and seeds if you have a history of kidney stones, as these foods are high in oxalates and may increase the risk of developing kidney stones.

Overall, nuts and seeds can be a healthy and nutritious addition to the diet of a pregnant woman, as long as they are consumed in moderation and as part of a balanced diet. It is a good idea to consult with a healthcare provider or a registered dietitian for personalized nutrition advice.

Oats

Oats are generally considered safe to eat during pregnancy. They are a good source of several essential nutrients, including fiber, protein, and various vitamins and minerals, which are important for fetal development and the health of the mother.

However, it is important to choose uncontaminated oats during pregnancy to reduce the risk of foodborne illness. Oats can be contaminated with harmful bacteria, such as Listeria, if they are grown in soil or processed in facilities that are not properly cleaned and maintained. It is a good idea to choose oats that are labeled as "certified pure" or "certified organic" to help ensure that they have been grown and processed in a clean and safe environment.

In addition, it is recommended to avoid consuming large amounts of oats or other high-fiber foods if you have a history of kidney stones, as these foods are high in oxalates and may increase the risk of developing kidney stones.

Overall, oats can be a healthy and nutritious addition to the diet of a pregnant woman, as long as they are properly prepared and consumed in moderation as part of a balanced diet. It is a good idea to consult with a healthcare provider or a registered dietitian for personalized nutrition advice.

Onigiri

Onigiri is a type of Japanese rice ball that is often filled with a variety of ingredients, such as vegetables, seafood, and meats. Onigiri can be a convenient and nutritious snack or meal option during pregnancy, as rice is a good source of energy and nutrients like B vitamins and iron. However, it is important to choose a variety of whole grains, including rice, during pregnancy to ensure adequate intake of these nutrients. It is also important to pay attention to the fillings used in onigiri, as some ingredients may not be suitable for pregnant women. For example, raw or undercooked seafood, meats, and eggs should be avoided during pregnancy due to the risk of foodborne illness. It is best to choose onigiri with cooked fillings or opt for a vegetable-based filling. It is also a good idea to check with a healthcare provider or a registered dietitian for individualized recommendations.

Onion rings

Onion rings are a popular snack or side dish made by coating thin slices of onion in a layer of breading and deep-frying them until crispy and golden brown. While onion rings can be a tasty treat, they are generally not considered a healthy or nutritious choice for pregnant women. Fried foods like onion rings are high in calories, fat, and added sugars, and should be consumed in moderation during pregnancy. It is important to maintain a balanced and varied diet during pregnancy, including a variety of fruits, vegetables, whole grains, and lean proteins. Instead of onion rings, it may be a better idea to choose healthier options like baked or grilled vegetables or whole grain snacks. It is also a good idea to check with a healthcare provider or a registered dietitian for individualized recommendations.

Onions

Onions are generally considered safe to eat during pregnancy. They are a good source of several essential nutrients, including vitamin C, potassium, and fiber, which are important for fetal development and the health of the mother.

However, it is important to follow proper food safety guidelines when consuming onions or any other produce during pregnancy. This includes washing the onions thoroughly to remove any dirt or contaminants, and discarding any onions that are spoiled or show signs of spoilage.

In addition, it is recommended to avoid consuming large amounts of onions or other high-fiber foods if you have a history of kidney stones, as these foods are high in oxalates and may increase the risk of developing kidney stones.

Overall, onions can be a healthy and nutritious addition to the diet of a pregnant woman, as long as they are properly prepared and consumed in moderation.

Onion rings

Onion rings are a popular snack or side dish made by coating thin slices of onion in a layer of breading and deep-frying them until crispy and golden brown. While onion rings can be a tasty treat, they are generally not considered a healthy or nutritious choice for pregnant women. Fried foods like onion rings are high in calories, fat, and added sugars, and should be consumed in moderation during pregnancy. It is important to maintain a balanced and varied diet during pregnancy, including a variety of fruits, vegetables, whole grains, and lean proteins. Instead of onion rings, it may be a better idea to choose healthier options like baked or grilled vegetables or whole grain snacks. It is also a good idea to check with a healthcare provider or a registered dietitian for individualized recommendations.

Oranges

Oranges are generally considered safe to eat during pregnancy. They are a good source of several essential nutrients, including vitamin C, folate, and potassium, which are important for fetal development and the health of the mother.

However, it is important to follow proper food safety guidelines when consuming oranges or any other produce during pregnancy. This includes washing the oranges thoroughly to remove any dirt or contaminants, and discarding any oranges that are spoiled or show signs of spoilage.

In addition, it is recommended to avoid consuming large amounts of oranges or other fruits if you are prone to developing gestational diabetes, as these foods are high in natural sugars and may increase the risk of developing this condition.

Overall, oranges can be a healthy and nutritious addition to the diet of a pregnant woman, as long as they are properly prepared and consumed in moderation.

Over-the-counter medications

It is generally not recommended to take over-the-counter (OTC) medications during pregnancy without consulting a healthcare provider first. Many OTC medications, including pain relievers, allergy medications, and cold and flu remedies, have not been tested for safety in pregnant women and may be harmful to the developing fetus.

Some OTC medications, such as acetaminophen (Tylenol) and ibuprofen (Advil), may be used cautiously during pregnancy under the guidance of a healthcare provider. However, it is important to avoid taking these medications in large doses or for long periods of time, as they can cause side effects and may be harmful to the developing fetus.

It is a good idea to consult with a healthcare provider before taking any OTC medications during pregnancy, and to follow the recommended dosage and frequency as directed. It is also a good idea to inform the healthcare provider about all medications, including OTC medications, that are being taken during pregnancy.

Overall, it is important to be cautious when taking OTC medications during pregnancy and to consult with a healthcare provider for personalized advice and guidance.

Oysters

Oysters are a type of shellfish that are often consumed raw or cooked. They are a good source of protein, iron, and other minerals, and may provide some health benefits. However, oysters can also carry certain risks for pregnant women. Raw or undercooked seafood, including oysters, can potentially contain harmful bacteria or parasites that can cause food poisoning. These risks can be higher during pregnancy, as the immune system is compromised and pregnant women are more susceptible to foodborne illness. It is important to be careful when consuming oysters or any other type of raw or undercooked seafood during pregnancy. It is best to avoid raw oysters or to ensure that they are thoroughly cooked before eating. If you are pregnant and considering consuming oysters or other raw or undercooked seafood, it is a good idea to consult with a healthcare provider or a registered dietitian for individualized advice.

Packaged snacks

Packaged snacks can be a convenient and tasty option for pregnant women, but it is important to choose snacks that are nutritious and safe to eat during pregnancy.

Some packaged snacks, such as crackers, pretzels, and rice cakes, can be a good source of whole grains and provide a moderate amount of nutrients. However, it is important to choose snacks that are low in added sugars, salt, and unhealthy fats, as these nutrients can contribute to weight gain and increase the risk of gestational diabetes and other pregnancy complications.

Other packaged snacks, such as chips, cookies, and candies, are generally not a good choice for pregnant women, as they are high in added sugars, salt, and unhealthy fats and provide little nutritional value. It is recommended to limit the intake of these types of snacks and choose healthier options instead.

In addition, it is important to follow proper food safety guidelines when consuming packaged snacks or any other food during pregnancy. This includes checking the expiration date and discarding any snacks that are spoiled or show signs of spoilage.

Overall, it is a good idea to choose packaged snacks that are nutritious and safe to eat during pregnancy, and to consume them in moderation as part of a balanced diet. It is a good idea to consult with a healthcare provider or a registered dietitian for personalized nutrition advice.

Pâté or meat spreads

Pâté or meat spreads can be a tasty and convenient snack option, but it is important to choose pâté or meat spreads that are safe to eat during pregnancy.

Some types of pâté, such as chicken liver pâté, can be high in vitamin A, which is important for fetal development but can be harmful to the developing fetus if consumed in excess. It is generally safe to consume small amounts of pâté or meat spreads that are made from poultry or cooked meats, but it is not recommended to consume large amounts or consume pâté or meat spreads that are made from raw or undercooked meats, as these can be contaminated with harmful bacteria, such as Listeria, which can cause serious illness or complications during pregnancy.

In addition, it is important to follow proper food safety guidelines when consuming pâté or meat spreads or any other food during pregnancy. This includes checking the expiration date and discarding any pâté or meat spreads that are spoiled or show signs of spoilage.

Overall, it is a good idea to choose pâté or meat spreads that are safe to eat during pregnancy and to consume them in moderation as part of a balanced diet. It is a good idea to consult with a healthcare provider or a registered dietitian for personalized nutrition advice.

Pancakes

Pancakes are a type of flat bread made from a mixture of flour, liquid, eggs, and leavening agents, such as baking powder or baking soda. They are typically cooked on a griddle or in a pan and can be served with a variety of toppings, such as syrup, butter, fruit, or chocolate chips. Pancakes can be a nutritious and delicious part of a well-balanced diet, provided they are made with whole grain flour and paired with nutritious toppings. However, it is important to be mindful of portion sizes and to choose ingredients that are safe for pregnant women.

Certain ingredients and toppings may not be suitable for pregnant women, such as raw eggs, raw or undercooked meats, and unpasteurized dairy products. It is also important to avoid added sugars and to choose whole grain flour, as refined flour may not provide as many nutrients as whole grain flour. If you are pregnant and considering consuming pancakes, it is a good idea to consult with a healthcare provider or a registered dietitian for individualized advice on what is safe and appropriate for you to consume.

Papaya smoothie

Papaya is a tropical fruit that is rich in vitamins, minerals, and antioxidants. It can be a healthy and refreshing addition to a pregnant woman's diet, especially when consumed as a smoothie.

Papaya is a good source of vitamin C, which is important for maintaining a healthy immune system and supporting the formation of collagen. It also contains a small amount of vitamin E, which is an antioxidant that can help protect cells from damage caused by free radicals. In addition, papaya is a good source of folate, which is an important nutrient for pregnant women as it helps to form the neural tube and can help prevent birth defects of the brain and spine.

While papaya is generally considered safe to consume during pregnancy, it is important to be mindful of the serving size. As with any food, it is best to consume papaya in moderation as part of a well-balanced diet. If you are pregnant and considering adding papaya to your diet, it is a good idea to speak with a healthcare provider or a registered dietitian for individualized guidance.

Pasta

Pasta is a type of food made from wheat flour, water, and sometimes eggs. It is a staple food in many cuisines and can be consumed in a variety of dishes, including sauces, soups, and casseroles. Pasta is a good source of energy, carbohydrates, and protein, and it can be a convenient and tasty option for pregnant women.

In general, pasta is considered safe to consume during pregnancy as long as it is cooked properly and consumed in moderation. It is important to choose whole grain pasta, which is made from whole grains and is higher in fiber and nutrients than refined pasta. Whole grain pasta can help to promote regular bowel movements, which can be helpful during pregnancy when constipation is common.

However, it is important to be mindful of the portion size and to balance pasta with other sources of nutrients, such as protein, fruits, and vegetables. It is also important to be aware of the sodium content of pasta sauces and to choose lower-sodium options if possible. If you have any concerns about consuming pasta during pregnancy, it is a good idea to speak with a healthcare provider or a registered dietitian for individualized guidance.

Pasta sauce

It is generally safe for pregnant women to consume pasta and pasta sauce. However, it is important to choose pasta and sauce made with whole grains, as they are more nutritious and can help to meet the increased energy and nutrient needs of pregnancy. It is also important to pay attention to portion sizes and to balance pasta with other nutrient-rich foods, such as vegetables, lean proteins, and healthy fats.

It is also important to be mindful of any added ingredients in pasta sauce, such as salt, sugar, and preservatives. It is generally recommended for pregnant women to limit their intake of added sugars and to choose sauces that are lower in sodium. Some types of pasta sauces, such as alfredo or carbonara, may also contain ingredients like cream or bacon that can be high in fat and should be consumed in moderation.

Overall, pasta and pasta sauce can be part of a healthy diet during pregnancy as long as they are consumed in moderation and balanced with other nutritious foods. It is always a good idea to consult with a healthcare provider or a registered dietitian for personalized nutrition advice during pregnancy.

Peaches

Peaches are generally considered safe to eat during pregnancy. They are a good source of several essential nutrients, including vitamin C, potassium, and fiber, which are important for fetal development and the health of the mother.

However, it is important to follow proper food safety guidelines when consuming peaches or any other produce during pregnancy. This includes washing the peaches thoroughly to remove any dirt or contaminants, and discarding any peaches that are spoiled or show signs of spoilage.

In addition, it is recommended to avoid consuming large amounts of peaches or other fruits if you are prone to developing gestational diabetes, as these foods are high in natural sugars and may increase the risk of developing this condition.

Overall, peaches can be a healthy and nutritious addition to the diet of a pregnant woman, as long as they are properly prepared and consumed in moderation.

Peanut butter

Peanut butter is generally considered safe to eat during pregnancy. It is a good source of protein, healthy fats, and various nutrients, including vitamin E, magnesium, and niacin, which are important for fetal development and the health of the mother.

However, it is important to choose peanut butter that is made from roasted peanuts and does not contain any added sugars, salt, or unhealthy fats. It is also a good idea to avoid consuming large amounts of peanut butter or any other high-fat foods if you are prone to developing gestational diabetes, as these foods can contribute to weight gain and increase the risk of developing this condition.

In addition, it is important to follow proper food safety guidelines when consuming peanut butter or any other food during pregnancy. This includes checking the expiration date and discarding any peanut butter that is spoiled or shows signs of spoilage.

Overall, peanut butter can be a healthy and nutritious addition to the diet of a pregnant woman, as long as it is consumed in moderation and as part of a balanced diet. It is a good idea to consult with a healthcare provider or a registered dietitian for personalized nutrition advice.

Peanuts

Peanuts are generally considered safe to eat during pregnancy. They are a good source of protein, healthy fats, and various nutrients, including vitamin E, magnesium, and niacin, which are important for fetal development and the health of the mother.

However, it is important to choose peanuts that are roasted or dry-roasted and do not contain any added sugars, salt, or unhealthy fats. It is also a good idea to avoid consuming large amounts of peanuts or any other high-fat foods if you are prone to developing gestational diabetes, as these foods can contribute to weight gain and increase the risk of developing this condition.

In addition, it is important to follow proper food safety guidelines when consuming peanuts or any other food during pregnancy. This includes checking the expiration date and discarding any peanuts that are spoiled or show signs of spoilage.

Overall, peanuts can be a healthy and nutritious addition to the diet of a pregnant woman, as long as they are consumed in moderation and as part of a balanced diet. It is a good idea to consult with a healthcare provider or a registered dietitian for personalized nutrition advice.

Pears

Pears are generally considered safe to eat during pregnancy. They are a good source of several essential nutrients, including vitamin C, potassium, and fiber, which are important for fetal development and the health of the mother.

However, it is important to follow proper food safety guidelines when consuming pears or any other produce during pregnancy. This includes washing the pears thoroughly to remove any dirt or contaminants, and discarding any pears that are spoiled or show signs of spoilage.

In addition, it is recommended to avoid consuming large amounts of pears or other fruits if you are prone to developing gestational diabetes, as these foods are high in natural sugars and may increase the risk of developing this condition.

Overall, pears can be a healthy and nutritious addition to the diet of a pregnant woman, as long as they are properly prepared and consumed in moderation.

Peas

Peas are generally considered safe to eat during pregnancy. They are a good source of several essential nutrients, including protein, fiber, and various vitamins and minerals, which are important for fetal development and the health of the mother.

However, it is important to follow proper food safety guidelines when consuming peas or any other produce during pregnancy. This includes washing the peas thoroughly to remove any dirt or contaminants, and discarding any peas that are spoiled or show signs of spoilage.

In addition, it is recommended to avoid consuming large amounts of peas or other high-fiber foods if you have a history of kidney stones, as these foods are high in oxalates and may increase the risk of developing kidney stones.

Overall, peas can be a healthy and nutritious addition to the diet of a pregnant woman, as long as they are properly prepared and consumed in moderation as part of a balanced diet. It is a good idea to consult with a healthcare provider or a registered dietitian for personalized nutrition advice.

Pecans

Pecans are generally considered safe to eat during pregnancy. They are a good source of healthy fats, protein, and various nutrients, including vitamin E, magnesium, and zinc, which are important for fetal development and the health of the mother.

However, it is important to choose unsalted pecans during pregnancy to help control sodium intake and reduce the risk of high blood pressure. It is also a good idea to avoid consuming large amounts of pecans or any other high-fat foods if you are prone to developing gestational diabetes, as these foods can contribute to weight gain and increase the risk of developing this condition.

In addition, it is important to follow proper food safety guidelines when consuming pecans or any other food during pregnancy. This includes checking the expiration date and discarding any pecans that are spoiled or show signs of spoilage.

Overall, pecans can be a healthy and nutritious addition to the diet of a pregnant woman, as long as they are consumed in moderation and as part of a balanced diet. It is a good idea to consult with a healthcare provider or a registered dietitian for personalized nutrition advice.

Peppers

Peppers are generally considered safe to eat during pregnancy. They are a good source of several essential nutrients, including vitamin C, potassium, and fiber, which are important for fetal development and the health of the mother.

However, it is important to follow proper food safety guidelines when consuming peppers or any other produce during pregnancy. This includes washing the peppers thoroughly to remove any dirt or contaminants, and discarding any peppers that are spoiled or show signs of spoilage.

In addition, it is recommended to avoid consuming large amounts of peppers or other high-fiber foods if you have a history of kidney stones, as these foods are high in oxalates and may increase the risk of developing kidney stones.

Overall, peppers can be a healthy and nutritious addition to the diet of a pregnant woman, as long as they are properly prepared and consumed in moderation as part of a balanced diet. It is a good idea to consult with a healthcare provider or a registered dietitian for personalized nutrition advice.

Pickled foods

Pickled foods can be a tasty and convenient snack option, but it is important to choose pickled foods that are safe to eat during pregnancy.

Some types of pickled foods, such as pickled vegetables, can be a good source of nutrients and provide a moderate amount of nutrients. However, it is important to choose pickled foods that are low in salt and added sugars, as these nutrients can contribute to high blood pressure and weight gain during pregnancy.

Other types of pickled foods, such as pickled eggs, pickled pigs' feet, and pickled herring, are generally not a good choice for pregnant women, as they can be high in salt and added sugars and provide little nutritional value. It is recommended to limit the intake of these types of pickled foods and choose healthier options instead.

In addition, it is important to follow proper food safety guidelines when consuming pickled foods or any other food during pregnancy. This includes checking the expiration date and discarding any pickled foods that are spoiled or show signs of spoilage.

Overall, it is a good idea to choose pickled foods that are nutritious and safe to eat during pregnancy, and to consume them in moderation as part of a balanced diet. It is a good idea to consult with a healthcare provider or a registered dietitian for personalized nutrition advice.

Pineapple

Pineapple is generally considered safe to eat during pregnancy. It is a good source of several essential nutrients, including vitamin C, potassium, and manganese, which are important for fetal development and the health of the mother.

However, it is important to follow proper food safety guidelines when consuming pineapple or any other produce during pregnancy. This includes washing the pineapple thoroughly to remove any dirt or contaminants, and discarding any pineapple that is spoiled or show signs of spoilage.

In addition, it is recommended to avoid consuming large amounts of pineapple or other fruits if you are prone to developing gestational diabetes, as these foods are high in natural sugars and may increase the risk of developing this condition.

It is also worth noting that pineapple contains an enzyme called bromelain, which can soften the cervix and potentially cause contractions. While the amounts of bromelain in pineapple are generally not high enough to cause problems during pregnancy, it is still a good idea to consume pineapple in moderation and to consult with a healthcare provider if you have any concerns.

Overall, pineapple can be a healthy and nutritious addition to the diet of a pregnant woman, as long as it is properly prepared and consumed in moderation.

Plums

Plums are generally considered safe to eat during pregnancy. They are a good source of several essential nutrients, including vitamin C, potassium, and fiber, which are important for fetal development and the health of the mother.

However, it is important to follow proper food safety guidelines when consuming plums or any other produce during pregnancy. This includes washing the plums thoroughly to remove any dirt or contaminants, and discarding any plums that are spoiled or show signs of spoilage.

In addition, it is recommended to avoid consuming large amounts of plums or other fruits if you are prone to developing gestational diabetes, as these foods are high in natural sugars and may increase the risk of developing this condition.

Overall, plums can be a healthy and nutritious addition to the diet of a pregnant woman, as long as they are properly prepared and consumed in moderation.

Prenatal vitamins

Prenatal vitamins are dietary supplements that are specifically designed for pregnant women to help meet the increased nutritional needs of pregnancy. These vitamins typically contain a variety of essential nutrients, including folic acid, iron, calcium, and various vitamins and minerals, which are important for fetal development and the health of the mother.

It is generally recommended for pregnant women to take a daily prenatal vitamin to help ensure that they are getting the nutrients they need during pregnancy. Prenatal vitamins can be an important part of a healthy pregnancy diet, but it is important to note that they are not a substitute for a balanced diet and should not be relied upon as the sole source of nutrients.

It is a good idea to consult with a healthcare provider or a registered dietitian to determine the best prenatal vitamin for your needs and to follow the recommended dosage and frequency as directed.

Overall, prenatal vitamins can be a helpful addition to the diet of a pregnant woman, but it is important to consume a variety of nutrient-rich foods and follow a balanced diet to meet the increased nutritional needs of pregnancy.

Processed foods

Processed foods are foods that have been altered in some way during preparation or storage. These foods may have had ingredients added or removed, or may have been treated with preservatives or other chemicals to extend their shelf life.

While some processed foods can be a convenient and tasty option, it is important to choose processed foods that are nutritious and safe to eat during pregnancy. Many processed foods, such as snack foods, frozen dinners, and fast foods, are high in added sugars, salt, and unhealthy fats and provide little nutritional value. These types of foods can contribute to weight gain and increase the risk of gestational diabetes and other pregnancy complications.

It is a good idea to limit the intake of processed foods during pregnancy and choose whole, unprocessed foods instead, as these foods are generally more nutritious and safer to consume. This includes a variety of fruits, vegetables, whole grains, lean proteins, and healthy fats, which are important for fetal development and the health of the mother.

In addition, it is important to follow proper food safety guidelines when consuming processed foods or any other food during pregnancy. This includes checking the expiration date and discarding any processed foods that are spoiled or show signs of spoilage.

Overall, it is a good idea to choose processed foods that are nutritious and safe to eat during pregnancy, and to consume them in moderation as part of a balanced diet. It is a good idea to consult with a healthcare provider or a registered dietitian for personalized nutrition advice.

Prunes

Prunes are generally considered safe to eat during pregnancy. They are a good source of several essential nutrients, including vitamin K, potassium, and fiber, which are important for fetal development and the health of the mother.

However, it is important to follow proper food safety guidelines when consuming prunes or any other produce during pregnancy. This includes washing the prunes thoroughly to remove any dirt or contaminants, and discarding any prunes that are spoiled or show signs of spoilage.

In addition, it is recommended to avoid consuming large amounts of prunes or other high-fiber foods if you have a history of kidney stones, as these foods are high in oxalates and may increase the risk of developing kidney stones.

Overall, prunes can be a healthy and nutritious addition to the diet of a pregnant woman, as long as they are properly prepared and consumed in moderation as part of a balanced diet. It is a good idea to consult with a healthcare provider or a registered dietitian for personalized nutrition advice.

Quiche

Quiche is a savory dish made with a pastry crust and a filling of eggs, milk or cream, and various other ingredients, such as vegetables, cheese, and meats. It is a popular breakfast, lunch, or dinner option that is enjoyed by people all over the world.

As a pregnant woman, it is generally safe to consume quiche. However, it is important to consider the ingredients and preparation methods used when deciding whether it is a suitable food for you. One of the main concerns with consuming quiche during pregnancy is the risk of foodborne illness. If the quiche is not handled or stored properly, it can harbor harmful bacteria, such as salmonella, that can cause serious illness. To minimize the risk of foodborne illness, it is important to follow proper food safety guidelines when preparing and storing quiche. This includes washing your hands thoroughly before handling food, keeping raw and cooked foods separate, and storing the quiche in the refrigerator to prevent the growth of harmful bacteria.

Another factor to consider when deciding whether to consume quiche during pregnancy is the nutritional content of the dish. Quiche is a good source of protein, which is important for the growth and development of the baby. However, it is also high in fat, sodium, and calories if made with high-fat ingredients, such as whole milk, cheese, and processed meats. To reduce the fat, sodium, and calorie content of quiche, it is a good idea to choose low-fat milk and cheese and healthy fillings, such as vegetables, lean meats, and beans. Quiche is also typically served with a variety of side dishes, such as salad or fruit, which can contribute to a balanced and nutritious diet.

Raisins

Dried raisins are a type of fruit that is made by drying grapes and removing their moisture content. Dried raisins are often sweetened with sugar or other sweeteners and may be used as a snack or as an ingredient in various types of recipes, such as baked goods or salads.

During pregnancy, it is generally considered safe to consume dried raisins as part of a healthy diet. Dried raisins are a good source of nutrients, including vitamins and minerals, and may have potential health benefits. Dried raisins may also be a good source of antioxidants, which may help to protect the body's cells from damage.

However, it is important for pregnant women to be aware of the potential risks of consuming dried raisins, as well as the potential benefits. Some pregnant women may be allergic to raisins or may have sensitivities to them. In addition, consuming large amounts of dried raisins may increase the risk of weight gain and other health problems due to their high sugar and calorie content.

It is generally recommended for pregnant women to consume dried raisins in moderation and to speak with their healthcare provider if they are concerned about the potential risks of consuming dried raisins. Pregnant women should also be aware of any food allergies or sensitivities they may have and should speak with their healthcare provider if they are concerned about the potential risks of consuming dried raisins.

Overall, dried raisins can be a tasty and convenient part of a healthy diet during pregnancy when consumed in moderation and with appropriate precautions. Pregnant women should speak with their healthcare provider about their dietary needs and any potential risks or concerns.

Red beans and rice

Red beans and rice is a traditional dish from Louisiana that is made with red beans, rice, and a variety of vegetables and spices. The red beans are typically cooked with a ham bone or other cured meats to add flavor and are served over a bed of rice. Red beans and rice is a popular meal option that is enjoyed by people all over the world.

As a pregnant woman, it is generally safe to consume red beans and rice. However, it is important to consider the ingredients and preparation methods used when deciding whether it is a suitable food for you. One of the main concerns with consuming red beans and rice during pregnancy is the risk of foodborne illness. If the red beans and rice are not handled or stored properly, they can harbor harmful bacteria, such as salmonella, that can cause serious illness. To minimize the risk of foodborne illness, it is important to follow proper food safety guidelines when preparing and storing red beans and rice. This includes washing your hands thoroughly before handling food, keeping raw and cooked foods separate, and storing the red beans and rice in the refrigerator to prevent the growth of harmful bacteria.

Another factor to consider when deciding whether to consume red beans and rice during pregnancy is the nutritional content of the dish. Red beans are a good source of protein, which is important for the growth and development of the baby. They are also a good source of fiber, which can help to prevent constipation, a common problem during pregnancy. Rice is a good source of complex carbohydrates, which provide energy and help to maintain blood sugar levels. However, it is important to note that the nutritional value of red beans and rice may depend on branding and other factors.

Rice

Rice is a type of grain that is widely consumed all over the world. It is a staple food in many cultures and is used in a variety of dishes, such as soups, stews, and casseroles. Rice is a good source of complex carbohydrates, which provide energy and help to maintain blood sugar levels. There are many types of rice, including white rice, brown rice, and wild rice, which differ in their nutritional content and taste.

As a pregnant woman, it is generally safe to consume rice. However, it is important to consider the type of rice and the method of preparation when deciding whether it is a suitable food for you. One of the main concerns with consuming rice during pregnancy is the risk of foodborne illness. If the rice is not handled or stored properly, it can harbor harmful bacteria, such as Bacillus cereus, that can cause serious illness. To minimize the risk of foodborne illness, it is important to follow proper food safety guidelines when preparing and storing rice. This includes washing your hands thoroughly before handling food, keeping raw and cooked foods separate, and storing the rice in the refrigerator to prevent the growth of harmful bacteria.

Another factor to consider when deciding whether to consume rice during pregnancy is the nutritional content of the grain. White rice is a refined grain that has been stripped of its bran and germ, which contain many of the grain's nutrients. As a result, white rice is not as nutritious as brown rice, which is a whole grain that contains the bran and germ. Brown rice is a good source of fiber, which can help to prevent constipation, a common problem during pregnancy. It is also a good source of vitamins and minerals, such as B vitamins, iron, and zinc. Wild rice is also a good source of nutrients, including protein, fiber, and B vitamins.

Overall, rice can be a safe and suitable option for pregnant women as long as it is prepared and stored safely and consumed in moderation. However, it is always a good idea to consult with a healthcare provider or a registered dietitian before making any significant changes to your diet during pregnancy. Every pregnancy is different, and what may be safe and suitable for one woman may not be the same for another. It is always a good idea to listen to your body and pay attention to any cravings or aversions you may have, as these can be a sign of your body's nutritional needs. In addition, it is important to follow a balanced and varied diet during pregnancy to ensure that you are getting all the nutrients you need for both your own health and the health of your baby.

Rice cakes

Packaged snacks can be a convenient and tasty option for pregnant women, but it is important to choose snacks that are nutritious and safe to eat during pregnancy.

Some packaged snacks, such as crackers, pretzels, and rice cakes, can be a good source of whole grains and provide a moderate amount of nutrients. However, it is important to choose snacks that are low in added sugars, salt, and unhealthy fats, as these nutrients can contribute to weight gain and increase the risk of gestational diabetes and other pregnancy complications.

Other packaged snacks, such as chips, cookies, and candies, are generally not a good choice for pregnant women, as they are high in added sugars, salt, and unhealthy fats and provide little nutritional value. It is recommended to limit the intake of these types of snacks and choose healthier options instead.

In addition, it is important to follow proper food safety guidelines when consuming packaged snacks or any other food during pregnancy. This includes checking the expiration date and discarding any snacks that are spoiled or show signs of spoilage.

Overall, it is a good idea to choose packaged snacks that are nutritious and safe to eat during pregnancy, and to consume them in moderation as part of a balanced diet. It is a good idea to consult with a healthcare provider or a registered dietitian for personalized nutrition advice.

Salsa

Quesadillas are a type of Mexican food made with tortillas filled with cheese and other ingredients, such as vegetables, meats, and beans. The tortillas are then grilled or heated until the cheese is melted and the quesadilla is warm. Quesadillas are a popular snack or meal option that is enjoyed by people all over the world.

As a pregnant woman, it is generally safe to consume quesadillas. However, it is important to consider the ingredients and preparation methods used when deciding whether they are a suitable food for you. One of the main concerns with consuming quesadillas during pregnancy is the risk of foodborne illness. If the quesadillas are not handled or stored properly, they can harbor harmful bacteria, such as salmonella, that can cause serious illness. To minimize the risk of foodborne illness, it is important to follow proper food safety guidelines when preparing and storing quesadillas. This includes washing your hands thoroughly before handling food, keeping raw and cooked foods separate, and storing the quesadillas in the refrigerator to prevent the growth of harmful bacteria.

Another factor to consider when deciding whether to consume quesadillas during pregnancy is the nutritional content of the dish. Quesadillas are typically made with tortillas, which are a good source of complex carbohydrates, which provide energy and help to maintain blood sugar levels. They also contain a variety of essential vitamins and minerals, such as iron, folic acid, and vitamin B6. However, it is important to note that the nutritional value of quesadillas may be limited due to the type of cheese and other fillings used. Quesadillas may be high in fat, sodium, and calories if made with high-fat cheese or processed meats, such as bacon or sausage. To reduce the fat, sodium, and calorie content of quesadillas, it is a good idea to choose low-fat cheese and healthy fillings, such as grilled chicken, vegetables, and beans.

In addition to the tortillas and fillings, quesadillas may also be served with a variety of toppings, such as salsa,

Sandwiches

A crispy chicken sandwich is a type of sandwich that typically consists of breaded and fried chicken that is served on a bun or other type of bread, along with various toppings, such as lettuce, tomato, cheese, and mayonnaise.

During pregnancy, it is generally considered safe to consume a crispy chicken sandwich as part of a healthy diet. Chicken is a good source of protein, which is important for the growth and development of the fetus and for the maintenance of the pregnant woman's tissues. Bread is a good source of carbohydrates, which provide energy to the body, and vegetables, such as lettuce and tomato, are a good source of nutrients, including vitamins and minerals.

However, it is important for pregnant women to be aware of the potential risks of consuming a crispy chicken sandwich, as well as the potential benefits. Some pregnant women may be allergic to chicken or may have sensitivities to it. In addition, consuming large amounts of fried foods may increase the risk of heart disease and other health problems.

It is generally recommended for pregnant women to consume a crispy chicken sandwich in moderation and to speak with their healthcare provider if they are concerned about the potential risks of consuming a crispy chicken sandwich. Pregnant women should also be aware of any food allergies or sensitivities they may have and should speak with their healthcare provider if they are concerned about the potential risks of consuming a crispy chicken sandwich.

Overall, a crispy chicken sandwich can be a tasty and convenient part of a healthy diet during pregnancy when consumed in moderation and with appropriate precautions. Pregnant women should speak with their healthcare provider about their dietary needs and any potential risks or concerns.

Sauces

Buffalo sauce is a spicy condiment that is made with hot sauce, vinegar, and other ingredients. While it can be a tasty addition to many dishes, it is important to choose buffalo sauce that is nutritious and safe to eat during pregnancy.

Many store-bought and homemade buffalo sauces are high in salt, added sugars, and unhealthy fats, and provide little nutritional value. These types of buffalo sauces can contribute to weight gain and increase the risk of gestational diabetes and other pregnancy complications.

It is a good idea to choose buffalo sauces that are made with healthier ingredients, such as hot sauce, vinegar, and minimal amounts of salt and unhealthy fats, and to limit the intake of added sugars and unhealthy fats. You can also make your own buffalo sauce at home using healthier ingredients, such as hot sauce, vinegar, and spices, to control the nutritional content of the sauce.

In addition, it is important to follow proper food safety guidelines when consuming buffalo sauce or any other food during pregnancy. This includes checking the expiration date and discarding any buffalo sauce that is spoiled or shows signs of spoilage.

Overall, it is a good idea to choose buffalo sauce that is nutritious and safe to eat during pregnancy, and to consume it in moderation as part of a balanced diet. It is a good idea to consult with a healthcare provider or a registered dietitian for personalized nutrition advice.

Caramel sauce is a sweet, smooth, and thick sauce that is made with caramelized sugar and other ingredients. While it can be a tasty addition to many dishes, it is important to choose caramel sauce that is nutritious and safe to eat during pregnancy.

Many store-bought and homemade caramel sauces are high in added sugars, salt, and unhealthy fats, and provide little nutritional value. These types of caramel sauces can contribute to weight gain and increase the risk of gestational diabetes and other pregnancy complications.

It is a good idea to choose caramel sauces that are made with healthier ingredients, such as natural sweeteners, and minimal amounts of salt and unhealthy fats, and to limit the intake of added sugars and unhealthy fats. You can also make your own caramel sauce at home using healthier ingredients, such as natural sweeteners and unsweetened milk or cream, to control the nutritional content of the sauce.

In addition, it is important to follow proper food safety guidelines when consuming caramel sauce or any other food during pregnancy. This includes checking the expiration date and discarding any caramel sauce that is spoiled or shows signs of spoilage.

Overall, it is a good idea to choose caramel sauce that is nutritious and safe to eat during pregnancy, and to consume it in moderation as part of a balanced diet. It is a good idea to consult with a healthcare provider or a registered dietitian for personalized nutrition advice.

Cranberry sauce is a type of condiment that is made with cranberries, sugar, and other ingredients and is often served with Thanksgiving or Christmas dinners. While it can be a tasty and convenient condiment option, it is important to choose cranberry sauce that is nutritious and safe to eat during pregnancy.

Many store-bought and homemade cranberry sauces are high in added sugars and calories, and provide little nutritional value. These types of cranberry sauces can contribute to weight gain and increase the risk of gestational diabetes and other pregnancy complications.

It is a good idea to choose cranberry sauce that is made with healthier ingredients, such as cranberries, natural sweeteners, and minimal amounts of unhealthy fats, and to limit the intake of added sugars. You can also make your own cranberry sauce at home using healthier ingredients, such as cranberries, natural sweeteners, and unsweetened fruit or nut butter, to control the nutritional content of the cranberry sauce.

In addition, it is important to follow proper food safety guidelines when consuming cranberry sauce or any other food during pregnancy. This includes checking the expiration date and discarding any cranberry sauce that is spoiled or shows signs of spoilage.

Overall, it is a good idea to choose cranberry sauce that is nutritious and safe to eat during pregnancy, and to consume it in moderation as part of a balanced diet. It is a good idea to consult with a healthcare provider or a registered dietitian for personalized nutrition advice.

Curry is a type of dish that is typically made with a blend of spices, herbs, and other ingredients and is often served with rice or other grains. Curry dishes may be made with a variety of meats, vegetables, and legumes, and may be flavored with various types of sauces or pastes.

During pregnancy, it is generally considered safe to consume curry as part of a healthy diet. Curry is a good source of nutrients, including vitamins and minerals, and may have potential health benefits. However, it is important for pregnant women to be aware of the potential risks of consuming curry, as well as the potential benefits.

Some pregnant women may be allergic to curry or may have sensitivities to it. In addition, consuming large amounts of curry may cause heartburn or other digestive problems in some individuals. Curry may also contain high levels of sodium or other ingredients that may not be suitable for pregnant women who are trying to manage their blood pressure or other health conditions.

It is generally recommended for pregnant women to consume curry in moderation and to speak with their healthcare provider if they are concerned about the potential risks of consuming curry. Pregnant women should also be aware of any food allergies or sensitivities they may have and should speak with their healthcare provider if they are concerned about the potential risks of consuming curry.

Overall, curry can be a flavorful and nutritious part of a healthy diet during pregnancy when consumed in moderation and with appropriate precautions. Pregnant women should speak with their healthcare provider about their dietary needs and any potential risks or concerns.

Sausage

Hot dogs are a type of processed meat, usually made from beef, pork, chicken, or a combination of these meats, that is formed into a sausage shape and cooked. Hot dogs are often served in a bun or roll and may be topped with a variety of condiments such as ketchup, mustard, onions, relish, cheese, and mayonnaise.

During pregnancy, it is generally considered safe to consume hot dogs as part of a healthy diet, as long as they are cooked to a safe temperature and handled properly to reduce the risk of food poisoning or other health problems. Processed meats like hot dogs are good sources of protein, iron, and other nutrients, which can be important for pregnant women.

However, it is important for pregnant women to be aware of the potential risks of consuming hot dogs, as well as the potential benefits. Some hot dogs may be high in sodium, added sugars, or other ingredients that may not be recommended for pregnant women in large amounts. In addition, consuming large amounts of hot dogs or other processed meats may increase the risk of certain health problems, such as heart disease or cancer.

It is generally recommended for pregnant women to consume hot dogs in moderation and to speak with their healthcare provider if they are concerned about the potential risks of consuming hot dogs. Pregnant women should also be aware of any food allergies or sensitivities they may have and should speak with their healthcare provider if they are concerned about the potential risks of consuming hot dogs.

Overall, hot dogs can be a tasty and convenient part of a healthy diet during pregnancy when consumed in moderation and with appropriate precautions. Pregnant women should speak with their healthcare provider about their dietary needs and any potential risks or concerns.

Seafood

It is generally recommended that pregnant women avoid consuming uncooked or undercooked meats, poultry, seafood, and eggs. This is because these types of foods can contain harmful bacteria that can cause foodborne illness.

Pregnant women are at increased risk of foodborne illness because their immune systems are compromised during pregnancy. Consuming undercooked or contaminated meats, poultry, seafood, or eggs can increase the risk of contracting a bacterial infection, such as salmonella or listeriosis. These infections can cause serious complications, including miscarriage, stillbirth, and severe illness in the mother.

To reduce the risk of foodborne illness, it is important for pregnant women to follow safe food handling practices, including:

- Washing hands thoroughly with soap and water before handling food
- Keeping raw meats, poultry, and seafood separate from other foods to prevent cross-contamination
- Cooking meats, poultry, and seafood to a safe internal temperature
- Avoiding raw or undercooked eggs
- Washing fruits and vegetables thoroughly before consuming

It is also important for pregnant women to be aware of the risks of consuming raw or undercooked foods and to choose cooked options instead. Pregnant women should also be cautious about consuming other types of raw or undercooked products, such as raw sprouts or unpasteurized milk and dairy products.

In summary, it is generally recommended that pregnant women avoid consuming uncooked or undercooked meats, poultry, seafood, and eggs to reduce the risk of contracting a bacterial infection. Pregnant women should follow safe food handling practices and choose cooked options instead.

Shellfish

It is generally recommended that pregnant women avoid consuming undercooked or raw shellfish. This is because shellfish can contain harmful bacteria and other contaminants that can cause foodborne illness.

Pregnant women are at increased risk of foodborne illness because their immune systems are compromised during pregnancy. Consuming undercooked or contaminated shellfish can increase the risk of contracting a bacterial infection, such as norovirus or Vibrio.

These infections can cause serious complications, including miscarriage, stillbirth, and severe illness in the mother.

To reduce the risk of foodborne illness, it is important for pregnant women to follow safe food handling practices, including washing their hands thoroughly with soap and water before handling food and cooking shellfish to a safe internal temperature. Pregnant women should also be cautious about consuming other types of raw or undercooked products, such as raw sprouts, uncooked or undercooked meats, poultry, seafood, and eggs, and unpasteurized milk and dairy products.

In summary, it is generally recommended that pregnant women avoid consuming undercooked or raw shellfish to reduce the risk of contracting a bacterial infection. Pregnant women should follow safe food handling practices and be cautious about consuming other types of raw or undercooked products.

Smoothies

Papaya is a tropical fruit that is rich in vitamins, minerals, and antioxidants. It can be a healthy and refreshing addition to a pregnant woman's diet, especially when consumed as a smoothie.

Papaya is a good source of vitamin C, which is important for maintaining a healthy immune system and supporting the formation of collagen. It also contains a small amount of vitamin E, which is an antioxidant that can help protect cells from damage caused by free radicals. In addition, papaya is a good source of folate, which is an important nutrient for pregnant women as it helps to form the neural tube and can help prevent birth defects of the brain and spine.

While papaya is generally considered safe to consume during pregnancy, it is important to be mindful of the serving size. As with any food, it is best to consume papaya in moderation as part of a well-balanced diet. If you are pregnant and considering adding papaya to your diet, it is a good idea to speak with a healthcare provider or a registered dietitian for individualized guidance.

It is generally safe for pregnant women to consume pineapple in moderation as part of a healthy and balanced diet. However, it is important to note that pineapple contains bromelain, which is a digestive enzyme that can soften the cervix and potentially cause early labor in high amounts. Therefore, it is generally recommended to avoid consuming large amounts of pineapple or pineapple supplements during pregnancy. It is also important to note that canned pineapple or pineapple juice may contain added sugars and preservatives, so it is best to opt for fresh pineapple whenever possible. As with any food or beverage, it is always a good idea to speak with a healthcare provider before making any significant changes to your diet during pregnancy.

Mango smoothies are a popular and refreshing beverage made with mango, milk, yogurt, and ice. They are often blended together until smooth and creamy and can be served cold or at room temperature. Mango smoothies can be a nutritious and enjoyable drink option, as long as they are made with safe and high-quality ingredients.

During pregnancy, mango smoothies can be a good source of nutrients such as protein, calcium, and vitamin D, which are important for pregnant women. Mango is also a good source of vitamin C, which is important for immune function and skin health.

However, it is important to be mindful of the type and quality of ingredients used to make mango smoothies, as some versions may be high in added sugars or other sweeteners. Pregnant women should choose mango smoothies made with low-fat or fat-free milk and yogurt, and minimal or no added sugars when possible. They should also be mindful of their intake of added sugars and should choose mango smoothies that are made with minimal or no added sugars when possible.

In addition, pregnant women should be aware of any food allergies or sensitivities they may have and should speak with their healthcare provider if they are concerned about the potential risks of consuming mango smoothies.

Overall, mango smoothies can be a nutritious and tasty drink option during pregnancy when consumed in moderation and with appropriate precautions. Pregnant women should speak with their healthcare provider about their dietary needs and any potential risks or concerns.

Snacks

Packaged snacks can be a convenient and tasty option for pregnant women, but it is important to choose snacks that are nutritious and safe to eat during pregnancy.

Some packaged snacks, such as crackers, pretzels, and rice cakes, can be a good source of whole grains and provide a moderate amount of nutrients. However, it is important to choose snacks that are low in added sugars, salt, and unhealthy fats, as these nutrients can contribute to weight gain and increase the risk of gestational diabetes and other pregnancy complications.

Other packaged snacks, such as chips, cookies, and candies, are generally not a good choice for pregnant women, as they are high in added sugars, salt, and unhealthy fats and provide little nutritional value. It is recommended to limit the intake of these types of snacks and choose healthier options instead.

In addition, it is important to follow proper food safety guidelines when consuming packaged snacks or any other food during pregnancy. This includes checking the expiration date and discarding any snacks that are spoiled or show signs of spoilage.

Overall, it is a good idea to choose packaged snacks that are nutritious and safe to eat during pregnancy, and to consume them in moderation as part of a balanced diet. It is a good idea to consult with a healthcare provider or a registered dietitian for personalized nutrition advice.

Soups

Broth is a type of liquid that is made by simmering bones, vegetables, and other ingredients in water. It is often used as a base for soups, stews, and other dishes. While broth can be a tasty and convenient ingredient, it is important to choose broth that is nutritious and safe to eat during pregnancy.

Many store-bought and homemade broths are high in salt, which can contribute to high blood pressure and other pregnancy complications. It is a good idea to choose broth that is low in salt or made with minimal amounts of salt, and to limit the intake of salt during pregnancy.

In addition, it is important to follow proper food safety guidelines when consuming broth or any other food during pregnancy. This includes checking the expiration date and discarding any broth that is spoiled or shows signs of spoilage.

Overall, broth can be a healthy and nutritious addition to the diet of a pregnant woman, as long as it is made with low-salt or minimal amounts of salt and consumed in moderation as part of a balanced diet. It is a good idea to consult with a healthcare provider or a registered dietitian for personalized nutrition advice.

Cream of mushroom soup is a type of soup that is made with mushrooms, milk or cream, and other ingredients and has a creamy and smooth texture. While it can be a tasty and convenient soup option, it is important to choose cream of mushroom soup that is nutritious and safe to eat during pregnancy.

Many store-bought and homemade cream of mushroom soups are high in unhealthy fats, added sugars, and sodium, and provide little nutritional value. These types of cream of mushroom soups can contribute to weight gain and increase the risk of gestational diabetes and other pregnancy complications.

It is a good idea to choose cream of mushroom soup that is made with healthier ingredients, such as mushrooms, low-fat or reduced-fat milk or cream, natural sweeteners, and minimal amounts of unhealthy fats and sodium, and to limit the intake of added sugars and unhealthy fats. You can also make your own cream of mushroom soup at home using healthier ingredients, such as mushrooms, low-fat or reduced-fat milk or cream, natural sweeteners, and unsweetened fruit or nut butter, to control the nutritional content of the cream of mushroom soup.

In addition, it is important to follow proper food safety guidelines when consuming cream of mushroom soup or any other food during pregnancy. This includes checking the expiration date and discarding any cream of mushroom soup that is spoiled or shows signs of spoilage.

Overall, it is a good idea to choose cream of mushroom soup that is nutritious and safe to eat during pregnancy, and to consume it in moderation as part of a balanced diet. It is a good idea to consult with a healthcare provider or a registered dietitian for personalized nutrition advice.

Soy sauce

High-sodium foods are foods that contain high levels of sodium, which is a type of mineral that is essential for the body's normal functioning. Sodium is found naturally in many foods, including meat, poultry, fish, and dairy products, and is also added to many processed and packaged foods to enhance flavor and extend shelf life.

During pregnancy, it is important for women to be aware of their sodium intake and to consume sodium in moderation. High levels of sodium intake during pregnancy can increase the risk of high blood pressure, which is a serious condition that can have negative effects on both the mother and the baby.

It is generally recommended for pregnant women to consume no more than 2,300 milligrams (mg) of sodium per day, which is the equivalent of about one teaspoon of salt. Pregnant women who are at risk of high blood pressure or who have pre-existing conditions such as diabetes may be advised to consume even lower levels of sodium.

Pregnant women should be aware of the sources of sodium in their diet and should aim to consume a variety of foods that are low in sodium. Examples of high-sodium foods that pregnant women should be cautious of include processed and packaged foods, such as canned soups, frozen dinners, and snack foods, as well as high-sodium condiments, such as soy sauce and salad dressings.

Spinach

Creamed spinach is a type of dish that is made by cooking spinach with cream or milk and is often served as a side dish or topping for other foods. Creamed spinach is a good source of nutrients, including vitamins, minerals, and antioxidants, and may have potential health benefits.

During pregnancy, it is generally considered safe to consume creamed spinach as part of a healthy diet. Spinach is a good source of nutrients that are important for the health and well-being of pregnant women, including vitamins K and C, folate, and potassium. Cream is a good source of nutrients, including proteins, fats, and vitamins, and may have potential benefits for certain health conditions, such as bone health and heart health.

However, it is important for pregnant women to be aware of the potential risks of consuming creamed spinach, as well as the potential benefits. Some pregnant women may be allergic to spinach or may have sensitivities to it. In addition, consuming large amounts of creamed spinach may cause heartburn or other digestive problems in some individuals.

It is generally recommended for pregnant women to consume creamed spinach in moderation and to speak with their healthcare provider if they are concerned about the potential risks of consuming creamed spinach. Pregnant women should also be aware of any food allergies or sensitivities they may have and should speak with their healthcare provider if they are concerned about the potential risks of consuming creamed spinach.

Overall, creamed spinach can be a nutritious and flavorful part of a healthy diet during pregnancy when consumed in moderation and with appropriate precautions. Pregnant women should speak with their healthcare provider about their dietary needs and any potential risks or concerns.

Sushi

Omega-3 fatty acid-rich foods, such as salmon, sardines, and walnuts, are generally considered safe to eat during pregnancy. Omega-3 fatty acids, which include EPA (eicosapentaenoic acid) and DHA (docosahexaenoic acid), are important for fetal brain and eye development and may also have other health benefits for the mother.

However, it is important to follow proper food safety guidelines when consuming omega-3 fatty acid-rich foods during pregnancy. This includes cooking fish thoroughly to reduce the risk of foodborne illness, and avoiding raw or undercooked fish, such as sushi or raw oysters, which can be contaminated with harmful bacteria.

In addition, it is recommended to avoid consuming large amounts of omega-3 fatty acid-rich foods if you have a history of allergies, as these foods can trigger allergic reactions in some people.

Overall, omega-3 fatty acid-rich foods can be a healthy and nutritious addition to the diet of a pregnant woman, as long as they are properly prepared and consumed in moderation as part of a balanced diet. The recommended daily intake of EPA and DHA during pregnancy is at least 200 mg per day. It is generally safe to consume up to 3,000 mg per day of EPA and DHA from foods, but it is not recommended to consume more than this amount. It is a good idea to consult with a healthcare provider or a registered dietitian for personalized nutrition advice.

Tacos

Guacamole is a popular Mexican dip or spread made from mashed avocados, diced onions, diced tomatoes, lime juice, and various herbs and spices. It is often served with tortilla chips or used as a topping for tacos, burritos, and other Mexican dishes.

During pregnancy, it is generally considered safe to consume guacamole as part of a healthy diet. Avocados are a good source of healthy fats, fiber, and various nutrients, including potassium, folate, and vitamin K. These nutrients can be important for pregnant women, as they may help to support fetal development and overall health.

However, it is important for pregnant women to be aware of the potential risks of consuming guacamole, as well as the potential benefits. Some guacamole recipes may contain raw onions or raw garlic, which can increase the risk of food poisoning or other health problems if they are not handled or prepared properly. In addition, guacamole may contain added sugars, sodium, or other ingredients that may not be recommended for pregnant women in large amounts.

It is generally recommended for pregnant women to consume guacamole in moderation and to speak with their healthcare provider if they are concerned about the potential risks of consuming guacamole. Pregnant women should also be aware of any food allergies or sensitivities they may have and should speak with their healthcare provider if they are concerned about the potential risks of consuming guacamole.

Overall, guacamole can be a tasty and convenient part of a healthy diet during pregnancy when consumed in moderation and with appropriate precautions. Pregnant women should speak with

their healthcare provider about their dietary needs and any potential risks or concerns.

Tofu

Lean proteins are types of protein that are lower in fat and calories compared to other types of protein and are often recommended as part of a healthy diet. Examples of lean proteins include chicken, fish, beans, and tofu.

During pregnancy, it is generally considered safe to consume lean proteins as part of a healthy diet. Lean proteins are a good source of nutrients that are important for the health and well-being of pregnant women, including protein, iron, and zinc. Protein is important for the growth and development of the fetus and for the maintenance of the pregnant woman's tissues, while iron is important for the production of red blood cells and for the transport of oxygen to the body's tissues. Zinc is important for the immune system, wound healing, and the sense of taste and smell.

However, it is important for pregnant women to be aware of the potential risks of consuming lean proteins, as well as the potential benefits. Some pregnant women may be allergic to certain lean proteins or may have sensitivities to them. In addition, consuming large amounts of certain lean proteins may cause heartburn or other digestive problems in some individuals.

It is generally recommended for pregnant women to consume lean proteins in moderation and to speak with their healthcare provider if they are concerned about the potential risks of consuming lean proteins. Pregnant women should also be aware of any food allergies or sensitivities they may have and should speak with their healthcare provider if they are concerned about the potential risks of consuming lean proteins.

Overall, lean proteins can be a nutritious and flavorful part of a healthy diet during pregnancy when consumed in moderation and with appropriate precautions. Pregnant women should speak with

their healthcare provider about their dietary needs and any potential risks or concerns.

Turkey

Deli meat, also known as luncheon meat or processed meat, is a type of meat that has been cured, smoked, or otherwise processed and is typically sliced thin and sold in a deli or grocery store. Deli meat includes a variety of products, such as ham, turkey, roast beef, and salami.

During pregnancy, it is generally recommended to avoid or limit the consumption of deli meat. Deli meat is often high in sodium, saturated fat, and other additives, which can increase the risk of certain health problems.

The World Health Organization (WHO) has classified processed meats, including deli meats, as a Group 1 carcinogen, which means that there is sufficient evidence to conclude that they are carcinogenic to humans. The WHO has also classified red meat, including beef, pork, and lamb, as a Group 2A carcinogen, which means that there is limited evidence to suggest that it may be carcinogenic to humans.

Pregnant women who are concerned about the potential health risks of consuming deli meat may want to consider limiting their intake of these products or choosing alternative sources of protein, such as poultry, fish, beans, and legumes.

It is important for pregnant women to speak with their healthcare provider about their dietary needs and any potential risks or concerns. Pregnant women should aim to follow a well-balanced diet that includes a variety of foods from all food groups, including protein-rich foods that are low in saturated fat and additives.

Vegetable broth

Broth is a type of liquid that is made by simmering bones, vegetables, and other ingredients in water. It is often used as a base for soups, stews, and other dishes. While broth can be a tasty and convenient ingredient, it is important to choose broth that is nutritious and safe to eat during pregnancy.

Many store-bought and homemade broths are high in salt, which can contribute to high blood pressure and other pregnancy complications. It is a good idea to choose broth that is low in salt or made with minimal amounts of salt, and to limit the intake of salt during pregnancy.

In addition, it is important to follow proper food safety guidelines when consuming broth or any other food during pregnancy. This includes checking the expiration date and discarding any broth that is spoiled or shows signs of spoilage.

Overall, broth can be a healthy and nutritious addition to the diet of a pregnant woman, as long as it is made with low-salt or minimal amounts of salt and consumed in moderation as part of a balanced diet. It is a good idea to consult with a healthcare provider or a registered dietitian for personalized nutrition advice.

Watermelon

Melons, such as watermelon and honeydew, are generally considered safe to eat during pregnancy. They are good sources of several essential nutrients, including vitamin C, potassium, and folate, which are important for fetal development and the health of the mother.

However, it is important to follow proper food safety guidelines when consuming melons or any other produce during pregnancy. This includes washing the melons thoroughly to remove any dirt or contaminants, and discarding any melons that are spoiled or show signs of spoilage.

In addition, it is recommended to avoid consuming large amounts of melons or other fruits if you are prone to developing gestational diabetes, as these foods are high in natural sugars and may increase the risk of developing this condition.

Overall, melons can be a healthy and nutritious addition to the diet of a pregnant woman, as long as they are properly prepared and consumed in moderation.

Yogurt (Mango Lassi)

Mango lassi is a refreshing and flavorful drink that is popular in South Asia and other parts of the world. It is made with mango, yogurt, milk, and ice, and is often blended together until smooth and creamy. Mango lassi can be served cold or at room temperature and is often enjoyed as a refreshing and hydrating beverage.

During pregnancy, mango lassi can be a nutritious and enjoyable drink option, as long as it is made with safe and high-quality ingredients. Mango lassi can be a good source of nutrients such as protein, calcium, and vitamin D, which are important for pregnant women. Mango is also a good source of vitamin C, which is important for immune function and skin health.

However, it is important to be mindful of the type and quality of ingredients used to make mango lassi, as some versions may be high in added sugars or other sweeteners. Pregnant women should choose mango lassi made with low-fat or fat-free yogurt and milk, and minimal or no added sugars when possible. They should also be mindful of their intake of added sugars and should choose mango lassi that is made with minimal or no added sugars when possible.

In addition, pregnant women should be aware of any food allergies or sensitivities they may have and should speak with their healthcare provider if they are concerned about the potential risks of consuming mango lassi.

Overall, mango lassi can be a nutritious and tasty drink option during pregnancy when consumed in moderation and with appropriate precautions. Pregnant women should speak with their healthcare provider about their dietary needs and any potential risks or concerns.

Zucchini (Lasagna)

Lasagna is a popular Italian dish made from layers of pasta, meat or vegetables, and cheese, typically baked in a casserole dish. Lasagna can be made with a variety of ingredients, including ground meat, vegetables such as zucchini or eggplant, and cheese such as mozzarella or Parmesan.

During pregnancy, lasagna can be consumed as part of a healthy and balanced diet, as long as it is prepared using safe food handling practices and cooked to a safe temperature. Lasagna can be a good source of protein, vitamins, minerals, and other nutrients, which can be important for pregnant women. However, lasagna may also contain ingredients that should be limited or avoided during pregnancy, such as high-fat meats, processed meats, and large amounts of cheese.

It is generally recommended for pregnant women to choose lean proteins, such as chicken, turkey, or tofu, and to limit their intake of high-fat meats and processed meats during pregnancy. Pregnant women should also be mindful of their intake of cheese and should choose low-fat or reduced-fat options when possible. Pregnant women should also be aware of any food allergies or sensitivities they may have and should speak with their healthcare provider if they are concerned about the potential risks of consuming lasagna.

Overall, lasagna can be a tasty and enjoyable part of a healthy diet during pregnancy when consumed in moderation and with appropriate precautions. Pregnant women should speak with their healthcare provider about their dietary needs and any potential risks or concerns.

MyPreggoPal.com

As an expectant mother, it's important to pay extra attention to your diet and ensure that you're getting all the nutrients you and your growing baby need. That's where MyPreggoPal can help. Our site is a one-stop-shop for all things pregnancy nutrition, with a wealth of information and resources to support you on your journey.

On MyPreggoPal, you'll find a variety of useful tools and resources, including:

- A week-by-week guide to pregnancy nutrition, with recommendations for each trimester
- A list of nutrients to focus on and foods to include in your diet, as well as those to avoid
- Delicious and healthy recipe ideas, with easy-to-follow instructions and nutrition information
- Tips for managing morning sickness and other common pregnancy discomforts
- A community forum where you can connect with other expectant mothers and share experiences and advice

In addition to all these resources, MyPreggoPal also offers a range of products and services to support you on your pregnancy journey. These include:

- One-on-one nutrition coaching with a registered dietitian
- Customized meal plans based on your specific needs and preferences
- A selection of pregnancy-specific supplements and vitamins
- Pregnancy-safe workouts and exercises to help you stay active and healthy

At MyPreggoPal, we believe that pregnancy is a special time in a woman's life, and we're here to support you every step of the way. So, if you're looking for reliable and expert-backed guidance on pregnancy nutrition, be sure to visit us at **mypreggopal.com**.

Thank You

Dear expectant mother,

I am grateful for your support in reading my book on pregnancy nutrition. As a student of medicine, I understand the importance of taking care of both your own health and the health of your growing baby. I hope that the information and resources provided in this book have been helpful to you on your pregnancy journey.

Writing this book has been a deeply personal and meaningful experience for me, and I am grateful for the opportunity to share my knowledge and insights with you.

Thank you for your interest in my work and for choosing to trust me as a source of information and support.

Sincerely,
Tavsimran S. Luthra

EATING FOR TWO: A GUIDE TO SAFE AND NUTRITIOUS CHOICES DURING PREGNANCY

www.ingramcontent.com/pod-product-compliance
Lightning Source LLC
Chambersburg PA
CBHW071218260726
48653CB00042B/1270